Nutrition and Fitness in Health and Disease

World Review of Nutrition and Dietetics

Vol. 72

Series Editor

Artemis P. Simopoulos, Washington, D.C.

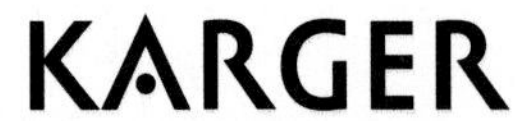

Basel · Freiburg · Paris · London · New York · New Delhi · Bangkok · Singapore · Tokyo · Sydney

2nd International Conference on Nutrition and Fitness, Athens, May 23–25, 1992

Nutrition and Fitness in Health and Disease

Volume Editor

Artemis P. Simopoulos

The Center for Genetics, Nutrition and Health,
American Association for World Health, Washington, D.C., USA

18 figures and 46 tables, 1993

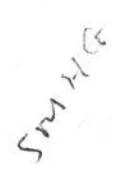

KARGER

Basel · Freiburg · Paris · London · New York · New Delhi · Bangkok · Singapore · Tokyo · Sydney

World Review of Nutrition and Dietetics

Library of Congress Cataloging-in-Publication Data
International Conference on Nutrition and Fitness (2nd : 1992 : Athens, Greece)
Nutrition and fitness in health and disease / 2nd International Conference on Nutrition and Fitness. Athens, May 23–25, 1992 ; volume editor, Artemis P. Simopoulos.
(World review of nutrition and dietetics ; vol. 72)
Includes bibliographical references and index.
1. Nutrition – – Congresses. 2. Nutritionally induced diseases – – Congresses.
3. Nutrition policy – – Congresses. 4. Physical fitness – – Congresses.
I. Simopoulos, Artemis P., 1933– . II. Title. III. Series.
[DNLM: 1. Diet – – congresses. 2. Nutrition – – congresses. 3. Physical Fitness – – congresses.]
ISBN 3–8055–5706–X (alk. paper)

Bibliographic Indices
This publication is listed in bibliographic services, including Current Contents® and Index Medicus.

Drug Dosage
The authors and the publisher have exerted every effort to ensure that drug selection and dosage set forth in this text are in accord with current recommendations and practice at the time of publication. However, in view of ongoing research, changes in government regulations, and the constant flow of information relating to drug therapy and drug reactions, the reader is urged to check the package insert for each drug for any change in indications and dosage and for added warnings and precautions. This is particularly important when the recommended agent is a new and/or infrequently employed drug.

Printed in Switzerland on acid-free paper by Thür AG Offsetdruck, Pratteln
ISBN 3–8055–5706–X

Contents

Panel V

Osteoporosis

Panel VI

New Concepts on Nutrition, Fitness and RDAs

Panel VII

Update on Policies and Programs in Nutrition and Physical Fitness

Panels I and II are published in volume 71 of this series.

Conference Organization

Organized by

The Center for Genetics, Nutrition and Health
The Hellenic Sports Research Institute (HSRI)
The Olympic Athletic Center of Athens, Spyros Louis

Under the Patronage of

The General Secretariat of Athletics of Greece – Ministry of Culture/International Olympic Academy (IOA)
Food and Agriculture Organization of the United Nations (FAO)
World Health Organization (WHO)

Sponsors

General Secretariat of Athletics of Greece
The President's Council on Physical Fitness and Sports, USA
Pan American Health Organization (PAHO)
National Institute of Child Health and Human Development, National Institutes of Health (NICHD-NIH)
Hellenic Pharmaceutical Association
International Union of Nutritional Sciences (IUNS)
American Association for World Health (AAWH)
Amway Corporation
Kellogg Company
'Slim Fast' Nutritional Foods International, Inc.

Additional Support for the Conference and the Proceedings Provided by

National Institute of Alcohol Abuse and Alcoholism, NIH
Mead Johnson Nutritional Group/Bristol-Myers
The NutraSweet Company
Eastman Chemical Products, Inc.
Henkel Corporation
McNeil Specialty Products Company
Campbell Soup Company

Honorary Chairman

Kyriakos Virvidakis, MD (Greece)

Executive Committee

Artemis P. Simopoulos, MD (USA), Chairman
Konstantinos N. Pavlou, ScD (Greece), Co-Chairman
Per-Olof Astrand, MD (Sweden)
George L. Blackburn, MD, PhD (USA)
Peter Bourne, MD (USA)
Ji Di Chen, MD (China)
Nicholas T. Christakos (USA)
J.E. Dutra-de-Oliveira, MD (Brazil)
Nikos Filaretos, IOA (Greece)
Frank Kotsonis, PhD (USA)
Eleazar Lara-Pantin, MD (Venezuela)
Alexander Leaf, MD (USA)
John Lupien (FAO)
Wim H.M. Saris, MD, PhD (The Netherlands)
Leonidas Seitanides, MD (Greece)
A. Stewart Truswell, MD (Australia)
Kihumbu Thairu, PhD (UK, Kenya)
Clyde Williams, PhD (UK)

Conference Planning Committee

Artemis P. Simopoulos, MD (USA), Chairman
Konstantinos N. Pavlou, ScD (Greece), Co-Chairman
George L. Blackburn, MD, PhD (USA)
Ji Di Chen, MD (China)
Carlos Hernan Daza, MD, PhD (PAHO)
J.E. Dutra-de-Oliveira, MD (Brazil)
Nikos Filaretos, IOA (Greece)
Eleni Grigoriadou, MD (Greece)
Anthony Kafatos, MD (Greece)
Demetre Labadarios, MD, PhD (South Africa)
Eleazar Lara-Pantin, MD (Venezuela)
Alexander Leaf, MD (USA)
John Lupien (FAO)
Evangelia Maglara-Katsilambrou (Greece)
Paul Nestel, MD (Australia)
York E. Onnen (USA)
Jana Pařízková, MD, PhD, DSc (Czechoslovakia)
Victor Rogozkin, DBS (Russia)
Leonidas Seitanides, MD (Greece)
Stamatis Skoutas, MD (Greece)
Kihumbu Thairu, PhD (UK, Kenya)
Clyde Williams, PhD (UK)

Hellenic Organizing Committee

Leonidas Seitanides, MD, President
Eustathios Matsoukas, MD, Vice President
Konstantinos N. Pavlou, ScD, Secretary
George Rontoyannis, MD, Treasurer

Members

Dimitrios Chasiotis, PhD
Eleni Grigoriadou, MD
Evangelia Maglara-Katsilambrou, RD
Antonios Kafatos, MD
Panagiotis Kontoulakos, MD
Panagiota Markou, RD
Stamatis Skoutas, MD
Panagiotis Stamatopoulos, MD
Alexandros Tsopanakis, PhD

Dedication

The proceedings of the conference are dedicated
to the concept of positive health as enunciated by the
Hippocratic physicians (5th century BC).

Positive health requires a knowledge of man's primary constitution
(which today we call genetics) and of the powers of various foods,
both those natural to them and those resulting from human skill
(today's processed food).
But eating alone is not enough for health.
There must also be exercise,
of which the effects must likewise be known.
The combination of these two things makes regimen,
when proper attention is given to the season of the year,
the changes of the winds,
the age of the individual and the situation of his home.
If there is any deficiency in food or exercise the body will fall sick.

Preface

This volume of World Review of Nutrition and Dietetics is the second volume of the proceedings of the Second International Conference on Nutrition and Fitness. The first volume of the proceedings (volume 71) consists of papers relevant to nutrition and fitness for athletes and the 46 abstracts from the poster session, whereas this volume consists of the papers relevant to the role of nutrition and fitness in health and disease and in growth and development throughout the life cycle.

In May 1988, the First International Conference on Nutrition and Fitness was held at the International Olympic Academy (IOA) at Ancient Olympia under the patronage of the International Olympic Committee (IOC) and the World Health Organization (WHO). It was considered most appropriate to hold the conference at Ancient Olympia because the importance of nutrition and physical fitness to health were first conceived in Greece and implemented at Ancient Olympia. The International Olympic Academy works under the auspices of the IOC as the only recognized Olympic academy. The IOA operates under the supervision of the Hellenic Olympic Committee for the promotion of the Olympic education. It is the spiritual center of the Olympic movement. Olympism is a concept with roots going back to ancient Greece; it contains fundamental aims for the education of man, and according to a phrase of Baron Pierre Coubertin, founder of the modern Olympic Games in 1896, 'Olympism tries to concentrate in a luminous beam all the principles that contribute to the perfection of man'. Ancient Greek philosophers believed that physical beauty, strength and health were not the only attributes men and women should have; however, when combined with moral and spiritual virtues and promoted through exercise and contests, these attributes can create a perfect man, a well-balanced being in all his elements and actions. Thus, through the academy, Olympia is the permanent center of Olympism and plans to widen its research work in parallel to its educational activities and participation of scientists from all disciplines. Thus, holding the First International Conference on Nutrition and Fitness reestablished nutrition as an important aspect of Olympism as it was in ancient times.

At the completion of the First International Conference on Nutrition and Fitness the following resolutions were made [1]:

(1) The participants of the conference wish to encourage governments to develop programs related to better nutrition and improved fitness.
(2) Nutrition policies should be coordinated with programs to improve physical fitness.
(3) Programs should take into consideration the variations in need in relation to different age groups and social circumstances for guidance about dietary needs and physical activity.
(4) IOC and WHO should be leaders in stimulating and providing guidance.
(5) We should meet in Olympia every 4 years before the Olympic games to update advice in the light of research results. We should continue to stimulate governments to develop and maintain programs on nutrition and fitness.

The Second International Conference on Nutrition and Fitness was held on May 23–25, 1992 at the Olympic Athletic Center of Athens 'Spyros Louis' under the patronage of the IOA, the Food and Agriculture Organization of the United Nations (FAO) and the World Health Organization (WHO). Seven hundred and eighty scientists and policy makers from academia, industry and government from 29 countries representing the 5 continents of Europe, Australia, North and South America, Asia and Africa attended the conference. The conference consisted of seven panels: Panel I: The Contribution of Macronutrients to Peak Performance of the Elite Athlete; Panel II: Concerns for Specific Population Groups in Relation to Nutrition and Fitness; Panel III: Diet and Exercise in Cardiovacular Disease; Panel IV: Obesity; Panel V: Osteoporosis; Panel VI: New Concepts on Nutrition, Fitness and RDAs; Panel VII: Update on Policies and Programs in Nutrition and Physical Fitness; and a special presentation on 'Exercise and Mood'.

The honorary chairman of the conference was Dr. Kyriakos Virvidakis, General Secretary of Athletics of Greece, who officially opened the conference and said that he was 'looking forward to the conference recommendations and the Declaration of Olympia on Nutrition and Fitness'. Dr. Virvidakis expressed his hope 'to see everyone again at the Third International Conference on Nutrition and Fitness in Greece'. Dr. Leonidas Seitanides, President of the Olympic Athletic Center of Athens, welcomed everyone and affirmed his belief in the concepts of nutrition and fitness being essential for health. John Lupien, Director of the Food Policy and Nutrition Division of the FAO said, 'In preparing for the International Conference on Nutrition (ICN) to be held in December 1992, FAO and WHO have become increasingly aware of the need for continued research into many different aspects of nutrition, dietary habits, exercise and lifestyles and the interrelationship between these factors. It is clear that the results of such research need wide dissemination and application and conferences of the type we are attending today are one of the most effective means to achieve this. In ICN preparation we have contacted many different organizations to obtain research information and different points of view to arrive at a consensus of the priority activities that need to be carried out in different countries. I look forward to hearing and participating in the presentations and deliberations on the many different aspects of nutrition and fitness which will take place in this conference over the next several days. I can assure you that the recommendations of this meeting will be a very timely addition to the ICN preparatory process and will be used in preparing the final ICN declaration and plan of action.'

Dr. Carlos Daza, representing WHO said, 'In this second International Conference, the World Health Organization is again pleased to grant its patronage to the International Conference on Nutrition and Fitness, jointly with the International Olympic Academy and the Food and Agriculture Organization of the United Nations. The first International Conference, held in Ancient Olympia in 1988, underlined the role of nutrition and fitness – as it was perceived by the Ancient Greeks – as part of the Olympic movement that has been for two millennia a vigorous stimulus for the physical and mental well-being of the human race. This Second International Conference on Nutrition and Fitness is highly relevant to the World Health Organization, for the member states are increasingly concerned about the ongoing nutrition and epidemiologic transitional trends, closely related to excessive or unbalanced dietary intake and sedentary habits. Both the objectives and topics of this conference are indeed relevant to WHO's priorities for healthy nutrition and lifestyle throughout the world, particularly with respect to the prevention of cardiovascular diseases, osteoporosis, obesity, cancer and functional consequences of erroneous diets and unhealthy behavior still affecting large groups of society. We look forward to the 'Declaration of Olympia on Nutrition and Fitness' as a corollary of this conference, based on the analysis of progress and accomplishments in nutrition and fitness made by your countries in the areas of research, training and program development. The World Health Organization is entirely willing to support renewed efforts and commitments of the international community and national governments to assure better nutrition for all people, reduction of hunger and malnutrition of vulnerable groups, elimination of micronutrient malnutrition and prevention of diet-related chronic and degenerative diseases'.

The conference cochairmen, Dr. Artemis P. Simopoulos and Dr. Konstantinos N. Pavlou thanked the conference participants and said that 'We will meet again in 1996, at which time we hope to have made considerable progress in having more countries participate in developing programs on nutrition and fitness'. This conference, as was the case with the first and all subsequent conferences, is dedicated to the concept of *positive health* as stated by the Hippocratic physicians.

Following the meeting in Athens, on May 26–27, 1992, a group of program participants from the Executive Committee and the Planning Committee representing Australia, Brazil, Greece, Kenya, Russia, South Africa, Sweden, UK, USA, Colombia and Venezuela, from the World Health Organization, the Pan American Health Organization, the Food and Agriculture Organization of the United Nations, the International Union of Nutritional Sciences, the Latin American Nutrition Society, the President's Council on Physical Fitness and Sports (USA), the Olympic Sports Center of Athens, The Center for Genetics, Nutrition and Health (USA), and other international organizations met at Ancient Olympia to develop the 'Declaration of Olympia on Nutrition and Fitness' [see pp. 1–8, this vol.].

As is customary, the group was welcomed by the representative of the IOA who officially opened the meeting with everyone listening to the Olympic hymn:

Immortal spirit of antiquity,
Father of the true, beautiful and good,
Descend, appear, shed over us thy light
Upon this ground and under this sky
Which had fits witnessed by unperishable fame.

Give life and animation to those noble games!
Throw wreaths of fadeless flowers to the victors
In the race and in the strife!
Create in our breasts, hearts of steel!

In thy light, plains, mountains and seas
Shine a roseate hue and form a vast temple
To which all nations throng to adore thee,
Oh immortal spirit of antiquity!

Official Olympic Hymn-Cantata by Costis Palamas
Set to Music by Spirou Samaras in 1896

The proceedings of the conference are published in two volumes in this series, volumes 71 and 72. Volume 71 is entitled 'Nutrition and Fitness for Athletes' and contains the papers from Panel I: The Contribution of Macronutrients to Peak Performance of the Elite Athlete; Panel II: Concerns for Specific Population Groups in Relation to Nutrition and Fitness; from Panel VI: New Concepts on Nutrition, Fitness and RDAs, the paper on 'Vitamin Requirements for Increased Physical Activity: Vitamin E'; from Panel VII: Update on Policies and Programs in Nutrition and Physical Fitness, the paper on 'Principles of Athletes' Nutrition in the Russian Federation'; the special presentation on 'Exercise and Mood'; and the conference poster abstracts. Volume 72 is entitled 'Nutrition and Fitness in Health and Disease' and contains the papers from Panel III: Diet and Exercise in Cardiovascular Disease; Panel IV: Obesity; Panel V: Osteoporosis; Panel VI: New Concepts on Nutrition, Fitness and RDAs; and Panel VII: Update on Policies and Programs in Nutrition and Physical Fitness.

The group felt strongly that the declaration of Olympia should be given wide distribution by having it published in major medical nutrition and sports journals in the languages of the participants. Everyone hoped that at the time of the Third International Conference on Nutrition and Fitness, many more countries will be participating and will have developed programs on Nutrition and Fitness.

These two volumes on nutrition and fitness should be of interest to practically everyone, but most definitely to physicians and scientists interested in the role of nutrition and fitness in health and performance, including nutritionists, exercise physiologists, geneticists, dietitians, educators, and policy makers (legislators and government officials).

Artemis P. Simopoulos, MD

Reference

1 Simopoulos AP (ed): Proceedings of the First International Conference on Nutrition and Fitness. Am J Clin Nutr 1989;49(suppl):909–1140.

Simopoulos AP (ed): Nutrition and Fitness in Health and Disease.
World Rev Nutr Diet. Basel, Karger, 1993, vol 72, pp 1–8

Declaration of Olympia on Nutrition and Fitness

May 26, 1992

The Second International Conference on Nutrition and Fitness met at the Olympic Athletic Center of Athens, May 23–25, 1992, under the patronage of the World Health Organization, the Food and Agriculture Organization of the United Nations, and the International Olympic Academy. Thirty-two scientific papers were presented to 780 registrants and 46 posters were displayed with results of recent investigations. A group of program participants met on May 26–27 at the International Olympic Academy, Ancient Olympia, to develop a declaration of aims and objectives resulting from the conference.

Present

Alexander Leaf (Cochairman), USA
Per-Olof Astrand (Cochairman), Sweden
Derek Prinsley (Secretary), Australia
Nicholas T. Christakos, USA
Carlos Hernan Daza, PAHO, WHO
Uri Goldbourt, Israel
Demetre Labadarios, South Africa
Eleazar Lara-Pantin, Venezuela
Meke Mukeshi, Kenya
J.E. Dutra-de-Oliveira, Brazil
York Onnen, USA
Konstantinos N. Pavlou, Greece
Eric Ravussin, USA (NIH)
Victor Rogozkin, Russia
Artemis P. Simopoulos, USA
Stewart Truswell, Australia
Clyde Williams, UK

Background

During the present century there have been unprecedented changes in life-style and patterns of health for humanity. Improved availability of wide varieties of food and less physical effort required for daily activities are prominent features of industrialized societies and of affluent groups in developing countries. However, humanity evolved during a more active, less-cushioned existence, with food often difficult to obtain. Present conditions in many affluent societies in which food choices are wide and physical activity is minimal may lead to poor nutrition with inadequate or incorrect food choices. Poor physical fitness results from a diminished need to be physically active. The interrelationship between nutrition and fitness is clear. The aims and objectives of the International Conference are to promote the advantages to health and fitness of good nutrition and regular physical activity for all stages of the human life span.

During more than 99% of our existence, human beings subsisted as hunters and food gatherers. During these 2 million years or more, our genetic code evolved to adapt us to a life-style as hunter-gatherers. Adaptations for survival were consonant with the need for habitual physical activity, including endurance and peak effort alternating with periods of rest and socialization. Major changes, however, have since taken place in both diet and physical activity. These changes began some 10,000 years ago with the development of agriculture and the domestication of animals. But increases in saturated fat from meat and dairy products, and trans fatty acids from margarines to present high levels, together with physical inactivity are much more recent phenomena, dating to the turn of this century. Even 10,000 years is too brief to allow significant adaptations to be made in our genetic code to these changes.

Human beings evolved on a diet that was not only low in saturated fats but was also balanced in the amounts of omega–6 and omega–3 fatty acids from seeds, green leafy vegetables, fish, and meat from animals and birds in the wild. The meat of wild animals and birds was lean, unlike the meat from domesticated, fattened cattle, sheep and fowl that human beings eat today. Thus, the diet was rich in vitamins and minerals and high in protein and fiber but low in fat. Vitamin C intake from wild green leafy vegetables and fruits was much higher than today's international recommendations and dietary allowances. The same was true for calcium and potassium, while the sodium content of the diet was lower than today's average intake.

Industrialized societies are characterized by an abundant and palatable food supply and by a sedentary existence at home, at work, and in transportation for most individuals. Today less than 1% of energy used in farm and factory work comes from muscle power, whereas at the beginning of this century some 30% of energy in these occupations came from human muscle power.

Children are naturally very active. They like to run and play, but today they are in schools (from nursery to kindergarten to primary and secondary schools) sitting most of the time. Few schools provide adequate programs or mandatory classes for physical exercise and individual involvement in sports. Instead, children have become spectators of sports rather than active participants in gymnastics, dance and informal play. Today the weight of a child may be predicted by the number of hours he or she watches television. Major increases in weight occur during adolescence and young adulthood with potentially dire consequences to health. Obesity is rampant in Western, developed societies and it is also occurring among the affluent in developing countries. Obesity is a major health problem of Western societies. It is apparently a health risk to change quickly from the life-style of a hunter-gatherer to that of a modern urban dweller. Insight into our biological heritage may help us to modify our current life-style in a positive way.

In most developing countries the nutritional problems are quite different. Dietary fat is already low and unrefined carbohydrate high but the intake of energy, protein, and micronutrients are all too often inadequate. A more bountiful and sanitary supply for all of the foods that are traditional in these cultures is needed. Surely, emulation of the excesses of the diets of Western, affluent societies is to be avoided.

We decry the existence of large numbers of hungry children and adults amidst the abundance of food in many of the industrialized countries. We call upon their governments to correct the maldistribution problems that allow such inhumane inequities to exist and to encourage food choices that provide optimal nutrition.

The Concept of Positive Health

In 480 BC, Hippocrates recognized the importance of the balance between food intake that provided fuel to the body (energy intake) and physical activity (energy expenditure) for health.

He developed the following concept of 'positive health':

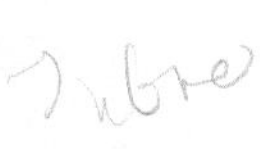

Positive health requires a knowledge of man's primary constitution (which today we call genetics) and of the powers of various foods, both those natural to them and those resulting from human skill (today's processed food). But eating alone is not enough for health. There must also be exercise, of which the effects must likewise be known. The combination of these two things makes regimen, when proper attention is given to the season of the year, the changes of the winds, the age of the individual and the situation of his home. If there is any deficiency in food or exercise the body will fall sick.

Hippocrates also noted that 'death occurs earlier in the obese'. In addition, the Olympic ideal emphasized the need to be responsible for one's body, and the belief that a healthy mind resides in a healthy body. Greeks were proud of their athletes, but gymnastics were part of everyone's daily activities, they were not just for the few. Among the Greeks, the concept of positive health was important and occupied much of their thinking. Those who had the means and the leisure applied themselves to maintaining positive health, conceived aesthetically as an end in itself.

The Olympic Ideal

From ancient times, sport in its most competitive form – the Olympic Games – has been regarded and practiced as a kind of art and has affected art in a special way. Sport as a noble emulation, stimulating continuous self-improvement and striving for the best performance of the competing athletes, had inevitably an aesthetic aspect and inspired the plastic arts: painting, pottery, sculpture and architecture, as well as poetry, music and literature. The Olympic spirit did not concern only perfection of bodily movement, but also the whole of the human being as a psychosomatic unit. The fundamental principle of the Olympic ideal was excellence, i.e. the athlete had to excel over others and over his own performance. Physical education with its forms of play and Greek agonistics were part of the culture of the time.

The setting of our conference and its follow-up in Ancient Olympia prompted recollections of the Olympic ideal of ancient Greece and the Hippocratic concept of positive health. Ideally, the concept of positive health should be related to each individual's genetic characteristics and environment together with adequate food and exercise. This principle of positive health should apply to all people, not just be limited to athletes and the affluent few. The appeal of a nutritional and physical fitness program should be broad, with particular attention directed to children. If such a program is to succeed, there will have to be increased training of health professionals in nutrition, exercise physiology and genetics.

To promote an optimal life-style and successful aging, an important and urgent challenge is to teach and promote good nutrition and regular physical activity from childhood to old age, including advice about smoking, alcohol abuse and other recognized threats to health. The message needs to be clear and then it becomes a matter of personal choice for a better quality of life that can be abetted by regular exercise and better-informed eating habits.

Children and Adolescents

Children are our future and their role and effectiveness in society will be directly related to their individual and collective physical and mental health. All children must have the opportunity to start life with a potential for fitness based on optimal health. To attain this goal, the following are needed.

(a) All expectant mothers should have access to proper prenatal care and counseling on the importance of smoking cessation and avoidance of alcohol and addictive drugs to optimize the prognosis for their offspring.

(b) All children should receive a healthful, nutritious diet without excesses or deficiencies of calories or essential nutrients. Instruction in nutrition and food should begin in childhood.

(c) All children should have the opportunity to engage in a variety of sports and physical fitness programs with emphasis on aerobic endurance, muscle strength, flexibility, and general fitness and to receive instruction in school about the health benefits of such exercise. Adoption of pleasurable forms of activity that can be enjoyed throughout life on a regular and frequent basis should be encouraged.

(d) All children and adolescents should be helped to avoid use of tobacco and abuse of alcohol and drugs and to abstain from early, unhealthful sexual practices.

(e) A positive self-image for all children should be fostered by universal access to education and opportunities to fulfill their potential in society.

(f) Universal access to health care should be provided for all children, with emphasis on primary care and health promotion to prevent illness and to achieve optimal health.

Promotion of good nutrition and regular aerobic physical activity for all throughout life must be a mainstay of any system that promotes the welfare of the individual and of society.

Physical Activity Improves Nutrition

Overweight due to excessive body fat is a major disorder of people in affluent and, increasingly, in some developing countries. Overweight increases the chance of developing chronic diseases including diabetes, high blood pressure, stroke, coronary heart disease, arthritis and possibly some forms of cancer. Ungainly appearance and reduced mobility hamper the individual's emotional well-being. Because obesity is often familial and has a strong genetic component, early identification of those at risk and proper counseling should aid in the prevention of obesity.

The two most effective measures to control overweight are regular physical activity and consumption of a low-fat diet. When people expend more energy through regular exercise and consume a wide variety of low-fat foods, the higher energy intake increases the probability that the resulting mixture of foods in their diet will meet requirements for all essential nutrients.

It should be emphasized that simple, nontaxing, physical activities, such as walking, cycling, swimming and gardening, are effective but must be regular, with a target of some such activity daily. Growing older in an environment where physical activity is encouraged and enjoyed can ensure continuation of such activities throughout life. Consequently, communities should be urged to provide opportunities and facilities particularly in cities, where open spaces and attractive worksite facilities will encourage physical activities for all age groups.

Performance

Good nutrition and regular physical exercise promote feelings of well-being and improve performance in all daily activities. For competing athletes energy intake must be adequate and consonant with levels of physical activity. Specific instruction is needed for adequate protein, high carbohydrate, low saturated fat, minerals, vitamin, and fluid intake. More research is needed on the nutritional requirements that will most effectively improve exercise capacity and performance.

Education, Development and Training

Because there is a dearth of training of health professionals in nutrition and physical education and a dereliction by them of responsibility for promoting this fundamental basis for good health, the public is bombarded by fads and conflicting pseudo-facts conceived by self-styled authorities. Information and education for the public is not provided in a reliable way. The opportunity for improved well-being through diet and physical activity is lost because the message has not been delivered effectively.

At present there is only minimal teaching in these disciplines of those who have educational and practical responsibilities for the health of the public. Therefore, there is a need to develop curricula in schools of nutrition, schools of physical education, and medical schools that will integrate nutrition, exercise physiology, and genetics into health education.

Declaration

(a) In developed countries technological developments have minimized physical activity, whereas variety and availability of foods make dietary choice a personal but not always well-advised decision.

(b) In most developing countries, the nutrition problems are quite different. Dietary fat is already low and unrefined carbohydrate high but the intake of energy, protein, and micronutrients are all too often inadequate. A more bountiful and sanitary supply of all the foods that are traditional in these cultures is needed. Surely, emulation of the excesses of the diets of Western affluent societies is to be avoided.

(c) The existence of large numbers of hungry children and adults amidst the abundance of food in many of the industrialized countries is destructive to the individual and to society. Governments must correct the maldistribution problems that allow such inhumane inequities to exist and encourage food choices that provide optimal nutrition for all.

(d) The adverse health effects of physical inactivity and consumption of high-fat diets have been repeatedly demonstrated in affluent societies by the high incidence of chronic diseases associated with these factors.

(e) Programs encouraging physical activity and good nutrition have now been shown to reduce diseases associated with inactivity and ill-advised diets, and can promote the quality of life.

(f) Understanding of the benefits to health from increased physical activity and good nutrition should be widely disseminated through extensive publicity.
(g) Health professionals should be educated in nutrition and exercise physiology to assume leadership roles in educating the public to the health benefits of physical activity and good nutrition.
(h) Education of the public should be promoted in schools at all levels, in the work place, through the media, and by health professionals.
(i) Advice provided to the public should be based on validated research findings in nutrition, genetics, and physiology. Research in these interrelated biomedical sciences deserves increased public and private support.
(j) Communities must provide clean and open spaces for children's playgrounds and adult sports and designate specific paths for pedestrians, cyclists, and other exercisers.
(k) Evidence is now convincing that general well-being and health can be greatly advanced by achievable adjustments of life-styles, nutrition, and physical activity. We call on all to respond.

Panel III
Diet and Exercise in Cardiovascular Disease

Simopoulos AP (ed): Nutrition and Fitness in Health and Disease.
World Rev Nutr Diet. Basel, Karger, 1993, vol 72, pp 9–22

Diet and Exercise in the Prevention of Cardiovascular Disease

George P. Rontoyannis[1]

Hellenic Sports Research Institute, Olympic Athletic Center of Athens,
'Spiros Louis', Athens, Greece

Introduction

Coronary heart disease (CHD) and essential hypertension are the most serious cardiovascular diseases in man in the Western World, influencing significantly morbidity and mortality.

Myocardial infarction remains the leading cause of death in various countries worldwide. In the USA, for instance, in 1981 out of about one million who died from cardiovascular diseases, almost two thirds died from CHD alone. About 4.6 million Americans were suffering from CHD. One fourth of a million who died from CHD were less than 65 years of age [1] and by the age of 60 years every 5th man and every 17th woman have already developed some form of CHD [2].

Arterial hypertension is another major public health problem, afflicting an estimated 15–30% of persons in most industrialized countries. It constitutes a leading risk factor for some other most prevalent and serious diseases such as CHD [3, 4] and stroke. Even mild hypertension contributes to the excess of cardiovascular disease morbidity and mortality [3, 5] as a result of its sequels CHD, stroke, and cardiac failure.

Treatment of established CHD, even under the most optimal conditions, can have only limited success in combating morbidity and mortality

[1] The author is very grateful to Dr. Christos Aravanis for his valuable suggestions in preparing the manuscript.

of the disease. Most important are the preventive measures that must be part of a national strategy to reduce this major health problem [6]. Indeed, the potential for prevention of cardiovascular disease is enormous. Long-term control of arterial hypertension, on the other hand, in persons with hypertension is of central strategic concern in the prevention of hypertension.

Primary prevention of cardiovascular disease is not only feasible but effective as well, particularly if it has started very early in life, and it is the best way to handle this serious health problem. This can be accomplished by reducing or eliminating existing, or even better, pre-existing risk factors. The total percentage of cardiovascular disease that is preventable by reducing risk factor exposure, to more nearly optimal level, may be calculated to be as much as 90%.

Diet and physical activity (exercise) are among the known effective means, together with changes in unhealthy habits (quitting cigarette smoking) or in behavior (shift from type A to type B personality), and the use of hypolipidemic drugs, in the primary and secondary prevention of cardiovascular disease.

Diet and exercise, considered separately or better, combined, have been shown to be effective in decreasing the magnitude of several major risk factors for cardiovascular disease, which are also predictors of this disease (table 1). All but family history, male sex and increasing age are modifiable cardiac risk factors [8].

The potential of diet regarding prevention of cardiovascular disease is enormous, since serum cholesterol, low-density lipoprotein cholesterol (LDLc), blood pressure, diabetes mellitus and obesity are clearly related to diet. Long-term dietary changes are effective, inexpensive and safe in lowering total cholesterol and LDLc levels in blood, and thus are important for primary and secondary prevention of CHD [9]. Dietary recommendations for the prevention of cardiovascular disease and a brief reference to intervention programs and suggestions follows later.

Physical activity, on the other hand, and movement in particular, is the fundamental attribute of the human machine, which is, from the phylogenetic and ontogenetic point of view, designed for movement [10] and has evolved biologically to perform daily, periods of continuous submaximal (aerobic) muscular activity, mainly walking [11]. For this reason the locomotor system is the biggest system of all other systems of the normal male adult accounting for 56–58% of his body weight [12] and a little less in women.

Table 1. Major risk factors for cardiovascular disease, coronary heart disease, cerebrovascular accident, and peripheral vascular disease in humans

Major risk factors	Role in atherogenesis	Modifiable by diet (D) and/or exercise (E)
Elevated total serum cholesterol	I (>200 mg/dl)	D, E
Elevated low-density lipoprotein	Pro, Po, Pre	D, E
Low high-density lipoprotein	Pro, Po, Pre	E, D
High level of triglycerides	Pro, Po, Pe	D, E
Hypertension	I, Pré	D, E
Cigarette smoking	I, Pro, Po, Pre	E (?)
Stress and type A personality	Pro, Po, Pre	E
Diabetes mellitus	I, Pro	D, E
Physical inactivity	Pro, Po, Pre	E
Obesity	Pro, Pre	D, E
Thrombotic tendencies	Po, Pre	E+D

Other risk factors are increasing age, positive family history, and male sex.
I = Initiator; Pro = promoter; Po = potentiator; Pre = precipitant.

Physical activity contributes to the existence and perfection of the human machine, ensuring anatomic integrity and functional efficiency not only of the locomotor, but also of all other systems. Finally, exercise, physical fitness and health are also interrelated.

Hippocrates, 25 centuries ago, recognizing the importance of balanced and healthy physical activity for the well-being of man, considered it as a major protective factor of his health and supplementary to medicine. According to Hippocrates, the aim of balanced and healthy physical activity is not to alter the health status but to preserve it, while medicine must change the condition of the diseased body to normal [13].

In the last decades several epidemiological studies have shown that leisure time regular physical activity (almost exclusively aerobic), during daily work or in transportation, can to a certain extent provide protection against cardiovascular diseases. The possible mechanisms through which exercise may confer protection from heart disease in man will be discussed.

Dietary Recommendations for Prevention of Cardiovascular Disease

Excessive energy intake and inappropriate eating habits have a major influence on the prevalence and incidence of atherosclerotic vascular disease. A few specific components of total nutrient intake define the atherogenic potential of a diet. High saturated fat, cholesterol and energy intake are uniformly associated with a higher blood cholesterol and higher frequency of myocardial infarction and death from CHD.

Consumption of saturated fats higher than 10% of the daily caloric intake is associated with high plasma cholesterol levels and increased atherosclerosis [14]. Cholesterol feeding or cholesterol restriction are related to increase or decrease in plasma cholesterol and the LDLc fraction, respectively. Severely hypercholesterolemic subjects are much more sensitive to dietary cholesterol than the normocholesterolemics [15]. In the last 10 years for populations in Western societies less than 100 mg/1,000 kcal of dietary cholesterol is recommended [16].

A total cholesterol level of 150 mg/dl that is possibly related with zero prevalence of significant coronary artery narrowing is determined as 'ideal' [8], while LDLc levels in plasma below 130 and 100 mg/dl are considered desirable and 'ideal', respectively. The LDLc/HDLc and total cholesterol/HDLc ratios, possibly the best indicators for CHD, 3.55/4.97 and 3.22/4.44 for males and females, respectively, may be sufficient dietary targets, since they are related to lower relative risk.

In some populations (American, Finnish, Dutch) dietary saturated fats accounted for 17–22% of total calories; in two Greek communities (Crete and Corfu) to about 7% and in some Japanese populations to less than 3% [14]. The current goal for the general population is to reduce saturated fats to less than 10% of calories, or even to 3%, when sufficient decrease in cholesterol and LDLc levels is recommended. Replacement of dietary saturated fats with unsaturated is necessary. In a population studied in Crete, where the lowest incidence rate (26/10,000) of CHD [17] among 16 populations from seven countries was found, almost 33% of total calories come from fats, 29% from the monounsaturated (mainly olive oil) and 3% from polyunsaturated fats [14], instead of the recommended 20% and about 7% of the calories, respectively [18].

Restriction of excessive calorie intake to keep body weight and fatness under control is important. Excess of body fatness (obesity), particularly that located in the abdominal and chest regions, is associated with higher LDLc levels in blood and increased risk of diabetes mellitus and hypertension. Inspiring individuals to eat less and to increase energy expenditure (exercise) is the only long-term course to weight control that is likely to be successful and healthy.

Adipose tissue less than 25 and 30% of body mass is considered 'prudent', while 16–19 and 19–22% is 'preferable' for adult males and females, respectively [19, 20]. The median sum of triceps and scapula skinfolds of the middle-aged male population studied in Crete [14] was only 14 mm, corresponding to less than 10% of body fatness. Alternatively, the 'ideal' body mass index is considered to be between 21 and 24.4 $kg \cdot m^{-2}$ and is related to the lower mortality rate [21, 22]. Body weight should not exceed 110% of the Metropolitan Life Insurance (1959) since this is the body weight which is not related with increased risk from cardiovascular disease [22].

Dietary characteristics that can play an important role in reducing the risk of arterial hypertension and maintaining blood pressure below 140/90 mm Hg are: low caloric, sodium and alcohol intake and possibly the relatively high consumption of potassium. Dietary salt of no more than 5 g/day is recommended [16].

Ultimate goals of nutrient intake for primary prevention of cardiovascular disease have been proposed in Europe [23] and in the USA [24], however for maximizing adherence to recommended dietary changes, it is preferable to have a phased approach to be followed and if possible to start it very early in life, shortly after the second year of age.

Intervention programs aimed at controlling cardiovascular disease with modification of diet have been found to be successful. However, as Pietinen et al. [25] stated: '... changing lifestyles in populations are a slow and not always a continuous process and the changes take place in stages; new ideas for intervention techniques are constantly needed and promotion of good nutrition and healther lifestyles in general calls for continuous efforts and food cooperation between researchers, health educators, legislators and food industry to make changes that are feasible for people.'

Two successful intervention dietary programs are worth mentioning. In Japan after a decrease in salt intake from 1960–1964 to 1980–1984, the mortality rate from cerebral strokes was decreased by 52% [26], and in Finland between 1972 and 1984, a decrease of fat and increase in fruit and vegetable consumption was paralleled with a significant decline of plasma cholesterol levels [25].

Intervention dietary programs, however, are not only useful in those populations with high prevalence of cardiovascular disease, but may be useful in those populations with low prevalence of this disease in order to keep it low. In Crete, for example, according to the Seven Countries Study coronary heart disease statistic rates, in 1960 in a rural male population they were found to have the lowest prevalence of CHD among 16 other populations [14]. However, an alarming situation has recently been revealed [27]. A dramatic increase in consumption of animal protein, fat and dairy products and a poor level of physical activity was recently found in an urban population sample of Crete; these changes were associated with an increase of almost 30% of the mean blood cholesterol levels [27]. These profound life-style changes call for measures aiming to persuade this population to re-establish traditional dietary patterns which is probably the prudent diet for prevention of cardiovascular disease, the Mediterranean diet. This traditional diet is mainly based on bread (380 g/day), potatoes (190 g/day), milk (235 g/day), fruits (464 g/day), vegetables (191 g/day), edible fats – mainly olive oil – (95 g/day), while its content in meat (35 g/day), and cheese (13 g/day) is relatively low, and the consumption of sweets is almost nil [28]. Monounsaturated fats (olive oil) have the best effects in keeping total serum cholesterol and LDLc low and at the same time in increasing HDLc.

Exercise and Cardiovascular Disease

Although a randomized trial on physical activity and primary prevention of CHD has not been accomplished successfully, and therefore no clear-cut proof is yet available that physical activity prevents cardiovascular disease, several epidemiological studies have shown that:

(a) Men engaged in vigorous physical activity in their leisure time with energy expenditure of up to 7.5 kcal/min may be protected to a certain level from fatal myocardial infarction or nonfatal coronary events, compared to inactive men [29].

(b) Men expending at work 8,500 or more calories per week had at any age significantly less risk of fatal coronary heart disease compared to men, whose job requires less muscular involvement [30].

(c) Former students engaged in energy expenditure of more than 2,000 kcal/week in leisure time activity showed a 39% less risk of CHD compared to those with less energy consumption rates. This indicates that vigorous exercise may be somewhat more protective than lighter activity [31].

(d) Even a low-level habitual physical activity at leisure time for more than 8 months per year is protective against acute coronary events [32].

Table 2. Possible mechanisms for preventing coronary artery disease or ischemic-related clinical consequences by aerobic exercise [based on ref. 37]

(a)	Retardation or regression of coronary arteries atherosclerosis, through 1 Control of related risk factors 2 Inhibition of clotting formation 3 Reduction of arterial wall cholesterol
(b)	Improvement of myocardial function through 1 Increase of myocardial capillaries, oxygen, delivery and/or utilization 2 Improvement of cardiac muscle efficiency, through increased contractility 3 Limitation of focal myocardial fibrosis
(c)	Reduction of ectopic ventricular activity

(e) An urban male population with relatively low physical activity has a higher (2.7 times) risk ratio to develop CHD than a rural population with higher muscular involvement [33].

(f) The protective effect of physical activity for the first infarction in males seems to be more significant in men with several major risk factors than in individuals with a low risk profile [34]. However, when hypercholesterolemia is high, as in the Finnish study, even the most intense sustained and regular muscular activity cannot protect sufficiently from CHD [35], indicating the limits of its potential in patients genetically predisposed to hypercholesterolemia.

In conclusion, active people develop CHD less frequently and more active persons have a lower risk for cardiovascular disease, but physical activity does not guarantee reduction of its incidence in those who are genetically predisposed, as it has been estimated that conversion from a sedentary to an active life style could eliminate 35% of CHD risk [36].

Aerobic exercise, which is the most appropriate exercise for improving aerobic capacity (main constituent of physical fitness in man), seems to be suitable for prevention of cardiovascular disease. Improvement of aerobic capacity is accomplished by an increase of maximal stroke volume and/or arteriovenous oxygen difference.

The possible mechanisms with which aerobic activity may confer protection from CHD and its clinical consequences may be related in delaying or even producing regression of arterial atherosclerosis with an improvement of myocardial function or a reduction of ectopic ventricular activity (table 2).

Table 3. Aerobic exercise to control major coronary risk factors and possible activated mechanisms

Coronary risk factors	Possible mechanisms activated	Characteristics of exercise – remarks
1 Dyslipidemias	a Increase of plasma FFA in circulation, through an increase in LPL activity (immediate effect) b Decrease of plasma TG levels (delayed effect) c Decrease of body fatness (delayed effect) d Increase of HDLc	For minimum efficiency walking, jogging, cycling, swimming at ~60% of maximum heart rate, 20 min per session, 3 times a week (~1,000 kcal/week). For optimum efficiency running, long-distance skiing, ball games, etc., at ~85% of maximum heart rate, 90 min per session, 7 times a week (~4,500 kcal/week), combined with isocaloric and balanced diet [38] and adjusted to the preferences of the exercising subjects; a prerequisite for a long-lasting program [39]. The exercise threshold stimulus for HDLc increase is equivalent to 18–20 km jogging per week and for long-term increase of HDLc with exercise (e.g. jogging) the weekly covered distance must exceed 42 km, that is required for improving aerobic capacity [40]. Vigorous and prolonged exercise for a long time period increases HDLc and the HDLc/LDLc ratio [41, 42], reduces body weight (fatness) [43] and promotes exogenous fat metabolism [44].
2 Arterial hypertension	a Reduction of resting cardiac output b Reduction of peripheral resistance c Increased sodium excretion in sweating and decreased body sodium content d Postexercise reduction of sympathetic tone e Postexercise relaxation f Decrease of body weight	Exercise intensity corresponding to 60–85% of maximum heart rate, with adjusted duration and frequency of repetition to achieve a weekly energy expenditure of ~14–20 $kcal \cdot kg^{-1}$ of body weight [45]. One hour of cycling, three times a week, with exercise intensity corresponding to the aerobic threshold reduces systolic blood pressure by ~15 mm Hg in hypertensive individuals [46]. Improvement of VO_2 max is negatively correlated with arterial blood pressure [47]. In clear contrast to the isotonic exercises isometric muscle contraction, especially when performed by small muscle groups, increase heart rate and blood pressure more than dynamic exercises do and linearly with age. Therefore, their intensity should not exceed 40–60% or 80% at most, of maximal voluntary contraction [48].

3 Obesity	a Invariable or decreased calorie intake, compared to energy consumed (inhibitory effect of exercise on calorie intake) b Decrease of body fatness due to increased rate of lipid utilization during mild or moderate exercise c Psychological enhancement while aerobic power and muscular strength are improving	Mainly aerobic exercise with energy expenditure $\geq$300 kcal/day, regularly performed by large muscle masses (e.g. walking, jogging, stair climbing, cross-country skiing, cycling, swimming) for a long period of time [49]. Three training sessions per week, including warming-up, aerobic exercise (walking-jogging: at first with an intensity ~70% of maximum heart rate and a mean distance covered per session ~2.4 km in about 22 min and walking-running later with an intensity ~85% of maximum heart rate and a mean distance covered per session 8.9 km in 46 min; various exercises – push-ups, sit-ups, knee flexion – extension, stretching) combined with low-calorie diet (~800 kcal/day) is most effective for mild obesity [50]. Physical activity for 30–60 min per session, repeated 2–5 times/week is usually well accepted by busy individuals [51].
4 Diabetes mellitus (or abnormal glucose tolerance test in normoglycemic middle-aged subjects)	a Improvement of glucose tolerance through 1 Increase in sensitivity and number of insulin receptors 2 Decrease of insulin requirements b Delayed atherosclerosis with control of related risk factors	Aerobic exercise of moderate intensity, 2 or more times per week [52], which corresponds to walking-jogging 25–35 km per week [53, 54] or to cycling [55]
5 Anxiety, stress	a Decrease of sympathetic tone b Improved physical appearance, self-confidence and mood c Temporary reduction of physical tension and anxiety	Aerobic exercise [56], with or without opponent, in pairs, undefined and general or competitive type [57, 58].

Optimum aerobic activity for delaying the onset of atherosclerosis has to be related to control of major cardiovascular risk factors. In table 3 clinically tested exercises are shown which are related to the control of dyslipidemias, arterial hypertension, obesity, diabetes mellitus, anxiety and stress, and the possibly activated mechanisms. These mechanisms are numerous and very different.

Although we do not know what is the threshold for cardiorespiratory fitness level in man that is correlated with sufficient protection from CHD, we assume that this level must not be very different from the level at which cardiorespiratory fitness begins to be considered 'good' for a middle-aged man. This level corresponds to about 40 ml of maximal oxygen consumption per kg of body weight per minute for men and somewhat less in women [20, 59].

Estimated energy expenditure during physical activity for minimum efficiency to control certain risk factors is about 150 kcal/day (about 1,000 kcal/week) and for maximum efficiency is about 650 kcal/day (about 4,500 kcal/week), while at about 300 kcal/day (≥2,000 kcal/week) certain protection from CHD is expected. These figures, however, must be considered relatively low compared to the estimated mean daily energy expenditure in the old way of farming of the male population studied in Crete [14], which seems to exceed 1,000 kcal/day.

Combined Diet and Exercise – Conclusions

Diet and exercise, according to existing information, are to a certain degree effective means by which to control major risk factors for cardiovascular disease, when used separately. Much better results can be achieved by their combined use. The synergistic effect of diet and exercise is seen in the treatment of dyslipidemias, in hypertension, in diabetes mellitus and in obesity. Exercise is an adjunct to diet.

Dietary intervention, for example, in elevated plasma LDLc in overweight people with restriction of calorie intake and decreased intake of saturated fats and cholesterol can reduce HDLc levels [60], which is undesirable. Combined, however, this kind of diet with regular exercise was shown recently [61] to be followed by an increase of HDLc together with a decrease in body weight and fatness.

In conclusion, the best pattern of combined diet and physical activity for the prevention of cardiovascular disease is, we suggest, that which is practiced in Crete. This pattern is associated with relatively very low prevalence of cardiovascular disease. Various aspects, however, for an ideally effective and safe combined diet and exercise pattern has to be further investigated. This pattern will be more effective if it will be practiced in a life-long period, in an aware and well-motivated population.

References

1 Kannel WB, Doyle JT, Ostfeld AM, Jenkins CD, Kuller L, Podell RN, Stamler J: Optimal resourses for primary prevention of atherosclerotic diseases. Atherosclerosis Study Group. Circulation 1984;70:157A–205A.
2 Castelli WP: Epidemiology of coronary heart disease: The Framingham study. Am J Med. 1984;76:4–12.
3 Stokes J, Kannel WB, Wolf PA, et al: Blood pressure as a risk factor for cardiovascular disease: The Framingham study –30 years of follow up. Hypertension 1989; 13(suppl I):113–118.
4 Roberts WC: Frequency of systematic hypertension in various cardiovascular diseases. Am J Cardiol 1987;60:1E–8E.
5 Stamler R, Neaton JD, Wentworth DN: Blood pressure (systolic and diastolic) and risk of fatal coronary heart disease. Hypertension 1989;13(suppl I):12–112.
6 Leaf A, Curfman GD: Introduction to preventive cardiology and cardiac rehabilitation. Cardiol Clin 1985;2:167–169.
7 Hopkins NP, Williams RR: Identification and relative weight of cardiovascular risk factors. Cardiol Clin 1986;1:3–31.
8 Castell N, Leaf A: Identification and assessment of cardiac risk. An overview. Cardiol Clin 1985;2:171–178.
9 Peters WL, Hegsted DM, Leaf A: Lipids, nutrition and coronary heart disease. Cardiol Clin 1985;2:179–191.
10 Meusel H: Developing physical fitness for the elderly through sport and exercise. Br J Sports Med 1984;March:4–12.
11 Astrand PO: Exercise and evolution; in: Exercise, Health and Medicine. Symposium Proceedings. British Sport Council and co-sponsors, May 3–6 1983, pp 11–12.
12 Cerretelli P: Fisiologia del lavoro e dello sport. Roma, Società Editrice Universo 1973, p 5.
13 Chrisafis JE: Gymnastics (γυμναστική) of Ancient Greeks (in Greek). Athens, National Acad Phys Educ Publ, 1965, p 69.
14 Keys A: Coronary heart disease in Seven Countries. Am Heart Assoc 1970;monogr 29:I162–I183.
15 Connor WE, Connor SL: The dietary treatment of hyperlipidemia. Med Clin North Am 1982;66:485–518.
16 James WPT: A European view of nutrition and emerging problems in the Third World. Am J Clin Nutr 1989;49:985–992.

17 Keys A: Seven Countries: A Multivariate Analysis of Death and Coronary Heart Disease. Massachusetts, Harvard University Press, 1980, p 319.
18 Brown WV: Dietary recommendations to prevent coronary heart disease, in Lee KT, Ondera K, Tanaka K (eds): Atherosclerosis. II. Recent Progress in Atherosclerosis Research. Ann NY Acad Sci 1990;376–388.
19 Bray GA: Overweight is risking fate. Definition, classification, prevalence and risks; in Wurtman RJ, Wurtman JJ (eds): Human Obesity. Ann NY Acad Sci 1987:14–28.
20 Cooper KH: The Aerobic Way. New York, Bantam Books, 1977, p 278.
21 Waaler HTh: Height, weight and mortality. The Norwegian experience. Acta Med Scand 1984;(suppl 679):1–56.
22 Simopoulos AP: Characteristics of obesity: An overview; in Wurtman RJ, Wurtman JJ (eds): Human Obesity. Ann NY Acad Sci 1987:4–13.
23 World Health Organization: Prevention of Coronary Heart Disease, Geneva; World Health Organization. 1982, Tech Rep Ser 678.
24 NIH Consensus Development Conference: Lowering Blood Cholesterol to Prevent Heart Disease. Washington, National Institutes of Health, 1984.
25 Pietinen P, Vartiainen E, Korhonen HJ, et al: Nutrition as a component in community control of cardiovascular disease (The North Karelia Project). Am J Clin Nutr 1989;49:1017–1024.
26 World Health Organization: World Health Statistics, Annual, Geneva, 1988.
27 Kafatos A, Kourounmalis I, Vlachonikolis I, Theodorou C, Labadarios D: Coronary heart disease: Factor status of the Cretan urban population in the 1980s. Am J Clin Nutr 1991;54:591–598.
28 Kromhout D, Keys A, Aravanis C, et al: Food consumption patterns in the 1960s in seven countries. Am J Clin Nutr 1989;49:889–894.
29 Morris JN, Everitt MG, Polland R, et al: Vigorous exercise in leisure-time: Protection against coronary heart-disease, Lancet 1980;ii:1207–1210.
30 Paffenbarger RS Jr, Hale WE: Work activity and coronary heart mortality. N Engl J Med 1975;292:545–550.
31 Paffenbarger RS Jr, Wing AL, Hyde RT: Chronic disease in former college students. XVI. Physical activity as an index of heart attack risk in college alumni. Am J Epidemiol 1978;108:161–175.
32 Magnus K, Matroos A, Strackee J: Walking, cycling, or gardening with or without seasonal interruption in relation to acute coronary events. Am J Epidemiol 1979; 110:724–733.
33 Garcia-Palmieri MR, Costas RJr, Cruz-Vidal M, et al: Increased physical activity: A protective factor against heart attack in Puerto-Rico. Am J Cardiol 1982;50:749–755.
34 Peters RK, Cady LD, Bischoff DP, et al: Physical fitness and subsequent myocardial infarction in healthy workers. JAMA 1983;249:3052–3056.
35 Punsar S, Karvonen MJ: Physical activity and coronary heart disease in populations from East and West Finland. Adv Cardiol 1976;18:196.
36 Paffenbarger RS, Hyde RT, Wing AL, Steinmets CH: A natural history of athleticism and cardiovascular health. JAMA 1984;252:491–495.
37 Oberman A: Exercise and the prevention of cardiovascular disease. Am J Cardiol 1985;55:10D–20D.

38 Tagarakis CBM, Rontoyannis GP: Lipids and exercise. (in Greek). Hippocrates 1989;2:143–153.
39 Wood PD: Dyslipoproteinemia; in Skinner J (ed): Exercise Testing and Exercise Prescription for Special Cases. Philadelphia, Lea & Febiger, 1987, pp 135–147.
40 Rogers MA, Yamamoto C, Hagberg JM, Holloszy JO, Ehsani AA: The effect of 7 years of intense exercise training on patients with coronary artery disease. J Am Coll Cardiol 1987;10:321–326.
41 Sallis JF, Haskell WL, Wood PD, Fortmann SP; Vranizan KM: Vigorous physical activity and cardiovascular risk factors in young adults. J Chron Dis 1986;39:115–120.
42 Goodyear LJ, Eronsoe MS, Honten DRV, Dover EV, Durstine JL: Increased HDL-cholesterol following eight weeks of progressive endurance training in female runners. Ann Sports Med 1986;3:33–38.
43 Sopko G, Leon AS, Jacobs DR Jr, et al: The effects of exercise and weight loss on plasma lipids in young obese men. Metabolism 1985;March:227–236.
44 Sady SP, Thompson PD, Cullinane EM, et al: Prolonged exercise augments plasma triglyceride clearance. JAMA 1986;256:2552–2555.
45 Gordon NF, Scott CB, Wilkinson WJ, Duncan JJ; Blair SN: Exercise and mild essential hypertension. Recommendations for adults. Sports Med 1990;6:390–404.
46 Urata H, Tanabe Y, Hiyonaga A, et al: Antihypertensive volume-depleting effects of mild exercise on essential hypertension. Hypertension 1987;9:245–252.
47 Saar E, Chayoth R, Meyerstein N: Physical activity and blood pressure in normotensive young women. Eur J Appl Physiol 1986;4:64–67.
48 Kobryn V, Hoffman B, Runsch E: Sex-and-related blood pressure response to dynamic work with small muscle masses. Eur J Appl Physiol 1986;4:79–82.
49 Gwinup G: Weight loss without dietary restriction: Efficacy of different forms of aerobic exercise. Am J Sports Med 1987;15:275–279.
50 Pavlou K, Steffe WP, Lerman RH, Burrows BA: Effects of diet and exercise on lean body mass oxygen uptake and strength. Med Sci Sports Exerc 1985;4:466–471.
51 Oscai LB: The role of exercise in weight control. Exerc Sport Sci Rev 1973;1:103–123.
52 Saltin B, Lingared F, Houston M, Horlin P, Hygaard E, Cad P: Physical training and glucose tolerance in middle-aged men and chemical diabetes. Diabetes 1979;(suppl 1):30–32.
53 Holloszy JO, Schultz J, Kusnierkiewicz J, Hagberg JM, Ehsani AA: Effects of exercise on glucose tolerance and insulin resistance: Brief review and some preliminary results. Acta Med Scand 1986;(Suppl 711):55–65.
54 Lampman RM, Santiga JT, Savage PJ, et al: Effect of exercise training on glucose tolerance, in vivo insulin sensitivity, lipid and lipoprotein concentrations in middle-aged men with mild hypertriglyceridemia. Metabolism 1985;March:205–211.
55 Rontoyannis GP, Druckenmiller M, Wangsness P, Nickolas C, Buskirk ER: Some effects of regular physical exercise in insulin dependent diabetics (in Greek with summary in English). Arch Med Soc 1983;9:136–144.
56 Raglin JS: Exercise and mental health. Beneficial and detrimental effects. Sports Med 1990;6:323–329.

57 Kranidiotis PT: The therapeutic value of sports activity in neurotic patients. Br J Sports Med 1973;(special issue):272–275.
58 Kranidiotis PT: Psychotherapeutic impact of physical activity and sport. (in Greek with summary in English). Athletiki Psicol 1984;2–3:19–29.
59 American College of Sports Medicine: Guideliness for Graded Exercise Testing and Exercise Prescription, ed. 2. Philadelphia, Lea & Febiger, 1980, p 52.
60 Krauss RM: Regulation of high density lipoprotein levels. Med Clin North Am 1982;6:403–430.
61 Wood PD, Stefanick ML, Williams PT, Haskell WL: The effects on plasma lipoproteins of a prudent weight-reducing diet with or without exercise, in overweight men and women. N Engl J Med 1991;325:461–466.

George P. Rontoyannis, MD, Hellenic Sports Research Institute,
Olympic Athletic Center of Athens, 'Spiros Louis', 37 Kifissias Avenue,
Athens 15123 (Greece)

Simopoulos AP (ed): Nutrition and Fitness in Health and Disease.
World Rev Nutr Diet. Basel, Karger, 1993, vol 72, pp 23–37

Coronary Heart Disease Prevention, Nutrition, Physical Exercise and Genetics: Rationale for Aiming at the Identification of Subgroups at Differing Genetic Risks

Uri Goldbourt[1]

Department of Epidemiology and Preventive Medicine, Sackler Medical School,
Tel Aviv University, Tel Aviv, Israel

Coronary heart disease (CHD) occurs at greatly varying rates in different countries. Moreover, pathological examination of atherosclerosis in a number of varied societies revealed a major ethnic and geographic variation [1]. Within single countries, ethnic diversity also abounds. Whites, Bantu and Indians in South Africa [2]; Lapps, Finns and Norsemen in Northern Norway [3]; Yemenite-born Jews and Jews originating from Europe in Israel [4], all differ greatly in their susceptibility to develop CHD.

Traditionally, we ascribe these differences, as well as differences between individuals within a cohort, to the coronary risk factors, such as blood levels of total and high-density lipoprotein cholesterol, blood pressure, cigarette smoking, diabetes mellitus, plasma fibrinogen, 'central' obesity, and physical inactivity. These risk factors are not fully independent. The degree of physical activity, for example, as well as diet, plays an important role in affecting the blood levels of lipids, the blood pressure and possibly the probability to develop diabetes mellitus via the effect of activity on body weight. Cigarette smoking considerably affects serum lev-

[1] Paper prepared during Sabbatical leave as Visiting Scientist with the Epidemiology and Biometry Program, Division of Epidemiology and Clinical Applications, National Heart, Lung and Blood Institute, NIH, Bethesda, Md., USA.

els of HDL cholesterol. Obesity affects the lipids, blood pressure and diabetes. In addition, the levels of the above factors (or the occurrence of diseases like diabetes that affect coronary risk) depend on both the genetic make-up of the individual and the effect of his/her behavior, lifestyle as well as of the physical environment and his/her close family environment.

Although a number of large prospective studies have demonstrated that knowledge of the main risk factors renders possible the identification of 20% of the population at risk, in whom about 50% or less of subsequent CHD will predictably occur [5–7], the rest of the disease burden will be found in individuals who are difficult to identify. This demonstrates that CHD incidence and, subsequently, CHD mortality vary above and beyond the 'explanatory variation' of risk factors. Our ability to accurately predict future CHD, on the basis of recognized risk factors, gradually diminishes with age [5]. The major reduction of CHD mortality in many of the developed countries [8] implies an increased age distribution of myocardial infarction (MI) patients, as the primary prevention of MI will result in increased age at first MI whereas the reduction of case fatality will bring many of the surviving patients to hospital with recurrent infarctions. Therefore, a preoccupation with 'premature CHD' is untimely. Cardiovascular epidemiology is increasingly becoming a geriatric discipline.

A major point to ponder is that apart from the insufficiency of the risk factors in fully discriminating those who will from those who will not develop CHD over a given period of time, not all the variation in the risk factors such as lipids, blood pressure, obesity or fibrinogen results from differences in eating, physical activity, work or familial stress or smoking, or other family and environmental conditions. A considerable portion of this variation actually stems from reasons that elude us. Increasingly, we realize that food, sedentary or active life habits, smoking, alcohol and drugs act on a background of highly variable individual constitutions. If we are to implement strategies of combating CHD, we have to better understand the underlying process, atherosclerosis of the coronary arteries [9]. We must also investigate and recognize what determines the levels of CHD risk factors in different individuals and what determines individual susceptibilities to the detrimental effects of the coronary risk factors.

On the basis of the strong evidence for the significant genetic component in CHD and in view of the topic of the conference in which this is presented, a goal of this paper is to review some new evidence that the individual responses to manipulation of the *diet as well as to physical*

Table 1. Occurrence of CHD in first-degree relatives of men from South and East Finland

Age at diagnosis of a first MI	Relative risk of having CHD by age 55[1]	
	South	East
Up to 45 years	11.4	6.7
46–50 years	8.3	3.6
51–55 years	1.3	1.8

[1] Risk of brothers of patients divided by risk of controls' brothers. Adapted from Rissanen [12].

exertion tend to vary on a genetic basis. An issue of immense public health significance is the definition of groups displaying differing risk, on the basis of genetic properties. If and when that can be done, thanks to the major advances in genetics and molecular biology, intervention programs, rather than being aimed in a sweeping manner at 'populations', would be targeted towards better defined groups at high risk. This will be discussed. Finally, I shall discuss new research avenues that, during the present decade, may provide us with important clues regarding the interaction of nutrition, genetics and environment in and its role in coronary disease.

Genetic Aspects of Coronary Heart Disease

The genetic aspects of CHD have been recognized for a number of decades and have been reviewed extensively [10, 11]. Perhaps the earliest aspect recognized was the familial aggregation of CHD. One of the original findings of Rissanen [12] in Finland indicated that CHD had been diagnosed 1.3 to 11 times as often in brothers of men with nonfatal MI as in brothers of disease-free matched controls, depending on the age of first MI. The latter was strongly associated with the probability of CHD in a brother. The findings held true in both the very high-incidence area of East Finland, at that time the territory with the highest known incidence internationally, as well as in the lower incidence part of the country (table 1). In 1982, ten-Kate et al. [13] demonstrated a 'net' twofold disease rate in first-degree relatives of patients. Nora et al. [14] indicated the existence of a stronger association between MI in the family and probability of CHD than was the case for any of the major risk factors. There is also ample evidence for the familial factors on the basis of comparing concordance rates in monozygotic and heterozygotic twins, histological findings in pathological investigation of coronary arteries in children and fetuses of different ethnic groups and from a number of other sources [10, 11]. The above evidence casts considerable doubt on the practice of distributing sweeping advice to populations, regardless of family history or other identifiable genetically determined differences in susceptibility to CHD.

Genetic Control of the Response to Dietary Regimens

A number of twin and adoptive studies have clearly established the influence of genetic factors in human obesity. The genetics of obesity are discussed in detail elsewhere in this issue [15]. Stunkard et al. [16] who studied the BMI of twins reared apart, found intra-pair correlation in the order of size of 0.7 and concluded that genetic influences on body mass are substantial. Genetic influences explained the majority of body mass variation, whereas as late as the 1970s it was felt that the balance of food intake and energy expenditure is fully or primarily responsible for body mass. Bouchard et al. [17] in the Physical Activity Science Laboratory at the Laval University in Quebec took this issue a decisive step further in their study of overfeeding of 12 MZ twins over 14 weeks, of which the excess calorie diet was given 6 days a week. The response to these 84,000 extra kcal exhibited overwhelming variation. Weight gains ranged between 4.3 and 13.3 kg over the study period. The most significant finding is the threefold variance *between* twin pairs as compared to that within. When gain in abdominal visceral fat, which is a more direct assessment of fat body mass gained, was assessed, the between-to-within variance ratio was as high as six (table 2). These results leave no doubt as to the role of genetics in determining body mass, fat mass and the response to overfeeding.

A volume of research supports the role of high blood concentration of LDL cholesterol as a promoter of atherosclerosis. The first of two large recent placebo control clinical trials seeking to alter the incidence of CHD by interfering with blood cholesterol levels, the Lipid Research Clinics Coronary Primary Prevention Trial (LRC-CPPT), demonstrated that the reduction of blood cholesterol levels in hypercholesterolemic middle-aged

Table 2. Effect of 100 days of overfeeding on trunk and abdominal fat, assessed by CT scan, in 12 pairs of male twins and the similarity within pairs in response to overfeeding

	CT-assessed fat, cm^2		Within-pair similarity adjusted for gain in fat mass	
	before overfeeding	after overfeeding	F ratio	interclass correlation
Trunk	250±99	448±107	3.8	0.58
Abdominal				
Total	106±46	199±50	4.1	0.60
Subcutaneous	72±40	141±46	3.8	0.58
Visceral	34±9	58±15	6.1	0.72

Adapted from Bouchard et al. [17]. F ratios are the ratios of variance between to variance within pairs and all are significantly >1 ($p < 0.05$, $p < 0.01$ for visceral and total abdominal fat).

subjects implied marked prognostic improvement in terms of subsequent coronary events [18]. Hence the importance of any means in the field of hygiene available for the control of blood cholesterol. National and international panels dealing with this problem have unequivocally recommended limits for the dietary intake of saturated fat and cholesterol [19]. These recommendations, however, fail to address the question whether all humans are alike in terms of their response to a dietary challenge of cholesterol and saturated fat. Katan and his group at Wageningen Agricultural University in the Netherlands have carried out a number of important experiments examining the effects of dietary saturated and unsaturated fatty acids and dietary cholesterol manipulation on blood lipids. In a sequence of three dietary trials [20] they divided the participants, on the basis of an initial response to a dietary load of cholesterol, achieved by manipulation of egg yolk intake, to putative hypo-, normo- and hyper-responders to cholesterol feeding. Despite the major limitation in individually identifying individuals on a basis of a single experiment, they went ahead to study the response of each of these groups to further experimentation. Thirty-two subjects participated in all three experiments; few exhibited declining serum cholesterol, whereas others reacted in varying degrees

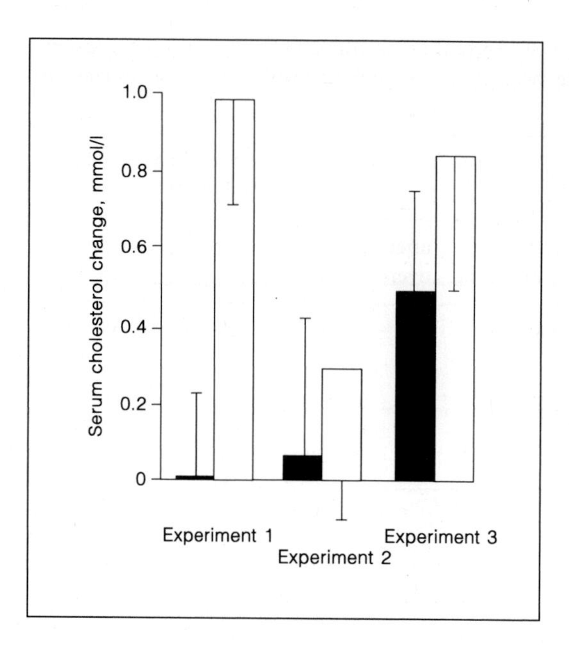

Fig. 1. Individuals with hypothetical hypo-, normo- and hyperresponse to cholesterol overfeeding and their reaction to successive dietary changes. Reprinted with permission from Katan et al. [20].

of cholesterol raising (fig. 1). In experiments 2 and 3, these groups continued to manifest major differences in their response to dietary cholesterol loading. Katan et al. concluded that differences in dietary response between humans are partly reproducible and are stable over a prolonged period. Thus, the concept of hypo- and hyperresponse, derived from animal studies where this phenomenon has been firmly established [21], has now found support in humans. They went further to study differences in responsiveness of serum cholesterol to dietary saturated fat and indicated a modest response variability [22], albeit accompanied by a tendency for the responses to dietary cholesterol and dietary saturated fat to be correlated [23]. Conversely, Grundy and Vega [24] who placed three groups under three regimens of unsaturated fatty acid substitution by saturated fat, indicate a marked individual variability in response to the latter. Interestingly, this occurred with almost identical response patterns among patients substituting saturated fat for high poly- or high monounsaturated fat. Intraindividual variability was not assessed in these participants, which may explain some of the differences between the Dutch and US studies. What appears to be lacking are investigations specifically designed to determine the range of responsiveness and which factors determine the variation.

The above examples demonstrate the interaction between genetics and nutrition, a topic likely to remain for some time at the focus of chronic disease research. A major aspect of this issue is whether, and to what extent, nutrients influence gene regulation and expression, an issue addressed in the 1989 Conference on Genetic Variation and Nutrition [25]. Nutritional factors regulated via dietary intake may interact with hormonal and other regulatory networks to regulate gene expression. The best known example in relation to CHD risk is the down-regulation of LDL receptor synthesis by increased dietary intake of saturated fat and cholesterol, a situation which is expressed in extreme in the inherited metabolic disorder known as familial hypercholesterolemia. Although in the latter disorder the removal of LDL from the blood is severely compromised, insufficient removal of LDL from the plasma can occur, to a lesser extent, in other individuals on a dietary basis. Brown and Goldstein, whose investigation of the LDL receptor is a landmark in both the genetics and the epidemiology of CHD, have therefore suggested that 'the human receptor system is designed to function in the presence of an exceedingly low LDL level' [26].

The basic mechanisms which underlie the influence of dietary factors and related metabolites on gene transcription are not well understood. The USA National Institutes of Health recently advanced proposals for support of investigations related to the mechanisms controlling gene regulation by dietary factors, as well as to the interaction between genetic factors and nutrition in general [27]. The proposal specifically encourages work on mechanisms influenced by hyper- and hypo-responsiveness to diet. The above discussion highlights the importance of such research in evaluating preventive efforts as well as dietary therapeutic regimen.

A timely example related both to the factors controlling response to a high fat diet and a possible dietary regulation of gene expression arises from a recently identified heritable lipoprotein phenotype. Evidence has been accumulating to suggest that circulating LDL particles can be described by two distinct phenotypes. The second of these two phenotypes, characterized by a predominance of small, dense particles, denoted as ALP (atherogenic lipoprotein type) B, is extremely common in the general population, perhaps as common as 30%. An autosomal-dominant mode of

Table 3. Effect of high fat versus low fat diet by atherogenic lipoprotein phenotype on lipo- and apolipoproteins (plasma level changes in mg/dl)

	'Stable A' (n = 51)	'Inducible A' (n = 36)	'Stable B' (n = 18)
Triglycerides	−20 ± 5	−60 ± 12	−60 ± 12
Total cholesterol	+12 ± 3	+16 ± 4	+24 ± 5
HDL cholesterol	+6 ± 1	+9 ± 1	+5 ± 1
LDL cholesterol	+10 ± 2	+19 ± 3	+30 ± 5
Apolipoprotein B	0 ± 2	−2 ± 2	+12 ± 3

inheritance has been indicated for ALP [28] and genetic linkage has been indicated between LDL subclass phenotypes and the LDL receptor on chromosome 19 [29]. Individuals with ALP B exhibit increased levels of serum triglycerides and low levels of HDL cholesterol (fig. 2). Each of these variables provides a significant discrimination between the two phenotypes. In an investigation designed to test whether the lipoprotein changes in phenotype B are responsive to changes in dietary fat intake, 105 men consumed, in random order, high fat (46%, 18% saturated) and low fat (24%, 6% saturated) diets, each for 6 weeks, with replacement of fat by carbohydrate. A constant polyunsaturated to saturated fat ratio as well as cholesterol and fiber intakes were maintained. The phenotype, determined by gradient gel electrophoresis, remained B on both diets in 15 men (stable B), A on both diets in 51 men (stable A) and fluctuated between A and B in 36 men [30, 31]. The high fat-low fat differences were threefold for LDL cholesterol, twofold for total cholesterol and threefold for triglycerides when the stable A and stable B groups were compared, with the differences for triglycerides expectedly inverse to those induced by dietary fat intake changes for cholesterol (table 3). The result may indicate both a considerably larger sensitivity of ALP type B to high fat in terms of its lipid response and a possible effect of the amount of fat on gene expression, a hypothesis that needs to be further studied. In the same group of men, 28 men with phenotype 4 of apolipoprotein E, a protein importantly involved in receptor-mediated uptake of LDL [32] (genotypes 3/4 and 4/4) exhibited a 24-mg/dl rise of total cholesterol under the high- as compared to the low-fat diet, significantly larger than that observed among counterparts with the 3/2 and 3/3 genotypes [31].

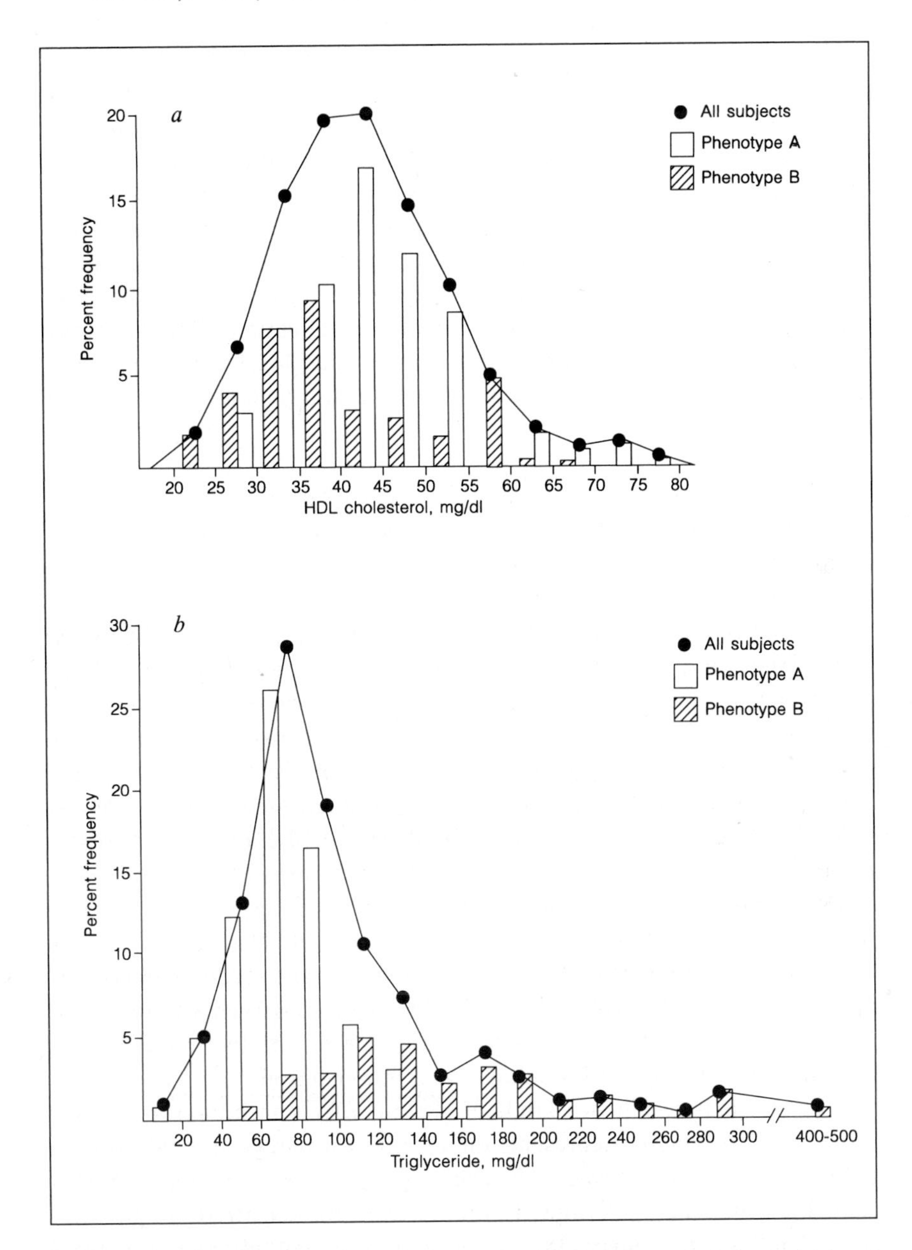

Fig. 2. Percent frequency distribution of adjusted plasma HDL cholesterol (*a*) and triglycerides (*b*) for 301 Mormons, by atherogenic lipoprotein phenotype. Adjustment is by covariance to the mean level for 50-year-old men. Reprinted with permission from Austin MA, et al: Atherogenic lipoprotein phenotype. Circulation 1990;82:495–506.

Non-lipid risk factors most probably vary in their response to dietary changes. Voluminous research has established the genetic sources of salt sensitivity and salt resistance. Thus, increased sodium intake may prove a significant insult to the maintenance of normal blood pressure in certain individuals but not others. Maternal-offspring resemblance in the change in blood pressure with salt restriction and phenotypes of haptoglobin possibly associated with salt sensitivity and resistance have been identified [33]. More comprehensive and accurate methods for identifying salt-sensitive individuals would have major preventive implications. Blood pressure response to dietary calcium may also be inherited [34]. Even taste perception is partly genetically determined [35]. Thus, genetics and nutrition interact in many ways.

Genetic Control of Human Energy Expenditure Components and the Response to Prolonged Exercise

The issue of genetic effects in determining the parameters of fitness and activity and the response to exercise owes, similar to research on inheritance of obesity, a great deal to the unique activities of the Laval University Research Group. In one of their experiments 11 MZ and 10 DZ twin pairs underwent a program of prolonged exercise [36]. The response of adipose tissue lipoprotein lipase (LPL) was assessed. The increase of LPL activity was very closely correlated within MZ and not as closely correlated within DZ twin pairs. Thus, adipose tissue LPL could be genetically determined in its basal activity as well as in response to exercise. Bouchard and Tremblay [37], in reviewing genetic effects in human energy expenditure components, indicated that a significant genetic component, approaching and perhaps surpassing 40% of the observed variance, had been demonstrated for the resting metabolic rate, the thermic effects of food and the energy cost for submaximal power output.

To summarize the two kinds of genetic effects in human metabolic properties: *Heritability* represents the extent to which genes contribute to the individual characteristics. The *genotype-environment interaction* represents the genetically determined differences in the sensitivity to environmental or lifestyle changes [38]. The gene-environment interaction is probably at the heart of human chronic disease development. Much of the genetic-epidemiologic approach to prevention would rest on identifying those with the 'bad genes' and teaching them how to avoid the hazardous effects of behaviors or environment that would prove uniquely damaging on their specific genetic background.

In the etiology of CHD we therefore have a complex network of associations, including genotype-environment interactions, that deserve to be better investigated and understood [10, 11]. The harnessing of recombinant DNA technology has paved the way to achieve just that. Recognizing the emerging importance of this field, the US National Heart, Lung and Blood Institute, Division of Epidemiology and Clinical Applications, has issued a proposal for a large Family and Genetic Study of Cardiovascular Disease (FGSCVD), intended as an investigation of heredity, lifestyles and behaviors that may influence the development of CHD and stroke. The long-term goals are to find new ways to prevent these diseases in high-risk families and in the general population. The study, coordinated by the Washington University Division of Biostatistics in Saint Louis, will involve the collection of *family* data in four US centers (the Minnesota and Chapel-Hill ARIC centers, The Utah Health Family Tree program and the Framingham Heart Study) where considerable research has already been done on individuals. The program will start with the ascertainment of 600 families on the basis of high-risk probands as well as of 600 control families, and represents the largest-scale effort in this field.

Rationale and Indications for Future Research and Preventive Strategies

Results from the Danish Adoption Register, published in 1988 [39], underscored a long-standing impression that both the environment, including household and cultural inheritance, and genetics play significant roles in the development of atherosclerosis and its sequelae. Table 4 demonstrates the importance of early death of either a biological parent or an adoptive parent in predicting adoptee mortality from vascular causes. This finding is notably absent in both cancer, where only the death of an adoptive parent predicted adoptee mortality from the same disease, and infectious diseases, where the reverse holds true.

Although history of fatal disease in biological parents, even though they did not share the same household with their offspring, is highly important in determining who is at high risk, and despite the well-recognized role of family history of CHD as an independent predictor of its incidence, intervention strategies recently devised in CHD are based on general rec-

Table 4. Risk of mortality in adoptees with at least one parent dead at age 50 relative to those whose parents were both alive at age 50 (RR); risks from causes concordant with biological or adoptive parents, Danish adoptees born 1924–1926

Cause of death		n	RR	95% confidence interval
All causes	Biologic	779	1.7	1.1–2.6
	Adoptive	913	0.7	0.4–1.4
'Natural causes'	Biologic	739	2.0	1.2–3.1
	Adoptive	889	1.0	0.5–1.9
Vascular disease	Biologic	585	4.5	1.3–15.4
	Adoptive	822	3.0	0.7–12.8
Cancer	Biologic	593	1.2	0.2–9.0
	Adoptive	818	5.2	1.2–22.2
Infectious disease	Biologic	641	5.8	2.5–13.7
	Adoptive	840	0.7	0.1–5.4

n = Number of parent-adoptee pairs included in the analysis. Adapted from Sorensen et al. [39].

ommendations to the public at large and on policies to detect, classify and treat individuals on the basis of a number of risk factors with insufficient emphasis on family history in particular and genetics in general. The available evidence strongly indicates that assessing the efficacy of preventive measures could be assisted by separate investigations of subgroups defined by stratification of genetic susceptibility [11]. This evidence justifies a major effort towards identification of *genetically characterized* subgroups at different underlying risks and at different underlying likelihoods to benefit from therapy. When this is achieved, even to a limited degree, recommendations should be reshaped. For example, families in which CHD has been frequent in successive generations, especially those where the biochemical, immunological or other physiological basis for the aggregation has been identified, should receive specific attention. As shown above, widely varying individual responses to lifestyle (dietary, exercise) intervention schemes probably represent genetically determined degrees of resistance to modifications of risk factor levels. The ultimate identification of such groups and the implementation of appropriate screening tests will facilitate the structuring of a *targeted* approach to find and help coronary prone families [40] and offer specific therapeutic advice to individuals. The search for genetic characteristics determining variability of risk factors and of their modifiability should therefore receive a high priority in pursuit of prevention of chronic diseases in general and CHD in particular.

References

1 McGill HC Jr, Arias-Stella J, Carbonelle LM, et al: General findings of the International Atherosclerosis Project. Lab Invest 1968;18:498–502.
2 Walker ARP: Studies bearing on coronary heart disease in South African populations. S Afr Med J 1973;47:85–90.
3 Thelle DS, Forde OH: The cardiovascular study in Finnmark county: coronary risk factors and the occurrence of myocardial infarction in first degree relatives and in subjects of different ethnic origin. Am J Epidemiol 1979;110:708–715.
4 Goldbourt U: Coronary Risk Factors and Cardiovascular Morbidity and Mortality among Yemenite-born Israeli Males in Comparison with Other Ethnic Groups. A Study in Genetic versus Environmental Susceptibility; PhD thesis, Tel Aviv University, 1983.
5 Kleinbaum DG, Kupper LL, Cassel JC, Tyroler HA: Multivariate analysis of risk of coronary heart disease in Evans County, Georgia. Arch Intern Med 1971;128:943–948.
6 Goldbourt U, Medalie JH, Neufeld HN: Clinical myocardial infarction over a 5-year period. III. Multivariate analysis of incidence. J Chron Dis 1975;28:217–237.
7 Heller RF, Chinn S, Tunstall-Pedoe HD, Rose G: How well can we predict coronary heart disease? Findings in the United Kingdom Heart Disease Prevention Project. Br Med J 1984;288:1409–1411.
8 Uemura K, Pisa Z: Recent trends in cardiovascular disease mortality in 27 industrialized countries. World Health Start Quart 1985;38:142–162.
9 Ross R: The pathogenesis of atherosclerosis: an update. N Engl J Med 1986;314: 488–500.
10 Berg K: Genetics of coronary heart disease; in Steinberg AG, Bearn AG, Motulsky AG, Childs B (eds): Progress in Medical Genetics, vol V. Philadelphia, Saunders, 1983, pp 36–90.
11 Goldbourt U, Neufeld HN: Genetic aspects of arteriosclerosis. Arteriosclerosis 1986;6:357–377.
12 Rissanen A: Familial occurrence of coronary heart disease in a high incidence area (North Karelia, Finland). Br Heart J 1979;42:294–303.
13 ten Kate LP, Boman H, Diger SP, Motulsky AG: Familial aggregation of heart disease and its relation to known risk factors. Am J Cardiol 1982;50:945–953.
14 Nora JJ, Lortscher RH, Spangler RD, Nora AH, Kimberling WJ: Genetic-epidemiologic study of early-onset ischemic heart disease. Circulation 1980;61:503–508.
15 Bouchard C: Genetics of obesity and its prevention; pp. 68–77, this volume.

16 Stunkard AJ, Harris JR, Pedersen NL, McClearn GE: The body-mass index of twins who have been reared apart. N Engl J Med 1990;322:1483–1487.
17 Bouchard C, Tremblay A, Despres J-P, Nadeau A, Lupien PJ, Theriault G, Dussault J, Moorjani S, Pinault S, Fournier G: The response to long-term overfeeding in identical twins. N Engl J Med 1990;322:1477–1482.
18 The Lipid Research Clinics Coronary Primary Prevention Trials: Results. I. Reduction in incidence of CHD. JAMA 1984;251:351–364.
19 Report of the National Cholesterol Education Program Expert Panel on Detection, Evaluation and Treatment of High Blood Cholesterol in Adults. Arch Intern Med 1988;148:36–69.
20 Katan MB, Beynen AC, deVries JHM, Nobels A: Existence of consistent hypo- and hyperresponders to dietary cholesterol in man. Am J Epidemiol 1986;123:221-234.
21 Eggen DA: Cholesterol metabolism in rhesus monkey, squirrel monkey, and baboon. J Lipid Res 1974;15:139–145.
22 Katan MB, van Gastel AC, de Rover CM, van Montfort NA, et al: Differences in individual responsiveness of serum cholesterol to fat modified diets in men. Eur J Clin Invest 1988;18:644–647.
23 Katan MB, Berns MA, Glatz JF, et al: Congruence of individual responsiveness to dietary cholesterol and to saturated fat in humans. J Lipid Res 1988;29:883–892.
24 Grundy SM, Vega GL: Plasma cholesterol responsiveness to saturated fatty acids. Am J Clin Nutr 1988;47:822–824.
25 Simopoulos AP, Childs B (eds): Genetic Variation and Nutrition. World Rev Nutr Dietetics, vol 63. Basel, Karger, 1990.
26 Brown MS, Goldstein JL: How LDL receptors influence cholesterol and atherosclerosis. Sci Am 1984;251:58–66.
27 NIH Guide, Volume 21, No 17, May 8, 1992.
28 Austin MA, King M-C, Vranzian KM, et al: Inheritance of low-density lipoprotein subclass patterns: Results of complex segregation analysis. Am J Hum Genet 1988; 43:838–846.
29 Austin MA, Krauss RM: Genetic control of low density lipoprotein subclasses. Lancet 1986;ii:592–595.
30 Dreon DM, Krauss RM: Low density lipoprotein subclass phenotypes are associated with differing lipoprotein responses to reduced fat diets. Circulation 1991; 84(suppl II): 681.
31 Krauss RM: Genetic factors affecting lipoprotein response to dietary fat. Presented at Genetics and Nutrition. Research Update and Policy Implications. Beltsville, Md, June 1992.
32 Davignon J, Gregg RE, Sing CF: Apolipoprotein E polymorphism and atherosclerosis. Arteriosclerosis 1988;8:1–21.
33 Luft FC, Miller JZ, Weinberger MH, Christian JC, Skrabal F: Genetic influences on the response to dietary salt, acute salt loading, or salt depletion in humans. J Cardiovasc Pharm 1988;12(suppl 3):S49–S55.
34 Mikami H, Ogihara T, Tabuchi Y: Blood pressure response to dietary calcium intervention in humans. Am J Hypertens 1990;3:147S–151S.
35 Miller IJ Jr, Reedy FE Jr: Variations in human taste bud density and taste intensity perception. Physiol Behav 1990;47:1213–1219.

36 Savard R, Bouchard C: Genetic effects in the response of adipose tissue lipoprotein lipase activity to prolonged exercise: A twin study. Int J Obesity 1990;14:771–777.
37 Bouchard C, Tremblay A: Genetic effects in human energy expenditure components. Int J Obesity 1990;14(suppl 1):49–55.
38 Bouchard C, Tremblay A, Nadeau A, et al: Genetic effect in resting and exercise metabolic rates. Metabolism 1989;38:364–370.
39 Sorensen TIA, Nielsen GG, Andersen PK, Teasdale TW: Genetic and environmental influence on premature death in adult adoptees. N Engl J Med 1988;318:727–732.
40 Williams RR: Nature, nurture, and family disposition. N Engl J Med 1988;318:769–771.

Uri Goldbourt, PhD, Neufeld Cardiac Research Institute, Sheba Medical Center, Tel Hashomer 52621 (Israel)

Simopoulos AP (ed): Nutrition and Fitness in Health and Disease.
World Rev Nutr Diet. Basel, Karger, 1993, vol 72, pp 38–48

Can Lifestyle Changes Reverse Coronary Heart Disease?

Dean Ornish

Preventive Medicine Research Institute, University of California, San Francisco, Sausalito, Calif., USA

Can Atherosclerosis Regress?

The Lifestyle Heart Trial is a randomized, controlled clinical trial to determine if ambulatory patients can be motivated to make and sustain comprehensive lifestyle changes and, if so, whether regression of coronary atherosclerosis can occur due to lifestyle changes alone. The Lifestyle Heart Trial is in two phases: phase 1 (after 1 year of intervention, completed), and phase 2 (the same patients after 4 years, still in progress).

Two previous trials in 1977 and 1980 assessed the short-term effects of lifestyle changes on coronary heart disease using noninvasive endpoint measures. Those two studies measured improvements in cardiac risk factors, functional status, myocardial perfusion [1], and left ventricular function [2].

In the Lifestyle Heart Trial, patients were randomly assigned to an experimental group asked to make comprehensive lifestyle changes or to a usual care control group who followed more conventional recommendations. Average percent diameter stenosis regressed from 40.0 to 37.8% in the experimental group yet progressed from 42.7 to 46.1% in the control group ($p = 0.001$). When only lesions greater than 50% stenosed were analyzed, average percent diameter stenosis regressed from 61.1 to 55.8% in the experimental group and progressed from 61.7 to 64.4% in the control group ($p = 0.03$). Overall, 82% of experimental group patients had an average change which was in the direction of regression. Degree of overall adherence was strongly related to changes in % diameter stenosis (%D) in a 'dose-response' relationship ($r = 0.62$, $p = 0.003$). Thus, comprehensive lifestyle changes may cause significant regression of even severe coronary atherosclerosis to begin occurring after only 1 year, whereas more moderate changes resulted in significant progression of atherosclerosis.

In the Lifestyle Heart Trial, patients with angiographically documented coronary artery disease at baseline who were not taking cholesterol-lowering drugs were randomly assigned to an experimental group or to a usual-care control group. All patients who were eligible and volunteered were accepted into the study. Experimental group patients were prescribed a lifestyle program that included a low-fat vegetarian diet, moderate aerobic exercise, stress management training, smoking cessation, and group support. Control group patients were not asked to make lifestyle changes although they were free to do so. Progression or regression of coronary artery lesions was assessed in both groups by quantitative coronary angiography at baseline and after approximately 1 year. Cine arteriograms made in San Francisco were sent to the University of Texas Medical School at Houston for quantitative analyses [3].

Patients completed a 3-day diet diary at baseline and after 1 year to assess nutrient intake and dietary adherence [4]. Patients were asked to complete a questionnaire describing smoking behavior and the type, frequency, and duration of exercise and of each stress management technique. Information from these adherence questionnaires was quantified using a formula determined a priori.

To reduce the possibility that knowledge of group assignment may bias the outcome measurements, the technicians responsible for all medical tests remained unaware of patient group assignment. Different personnel provided the lifestyle intervention, performed the tests, analyzed the results, and computed statistical analyses.

Experimental-group patients were asked to consume a low-fat vegetarian diet for at least 1 year. The diet included fruits, vegetables, grains, legumes, and soybean products without caloric restriction. No animal products were allowed except for egg whites and one cup per day of non-fat milk or yogurt. The diet contained approximately 10% of calories as fat (P/S ratio >1), 15–20% protein, and 70–75% predominantly complex carbohydrates. Cholesterol intake was limited to 5 mg/day or less. Salt was restricted only for hypertensive patients. Caffeine was eliminated, and alcohol was limited to no more than 2 ounces per day or equivalent. The stress management techniques included stretching exercises, breathing techniques, meditation, progressive relaxation, and imagery [5–8]. Patients were asked to practice these stress management techniques for at least one hour per day. Patients were individually prescribed exercise levels (typically walking) according to their baseline treadmill test results. Patients were asked to exercise for a minimum of three hours per week and to spend a minimum of 30 min per session exercising within their target heart rates. The twice-weekly group discussions provided social support to help patients adhere to the lifestyle-change program [9].

Differences in baseline characteristics of experimental and control group patients were tested for statistical significance by use of conventional t-tests. Comparisons of these two study groups with respect to baseline coronary artery lesion characteristics (measured by quantitative coronary angiography) and changes in lesion characteristics from pre- to post-intervention were examined via a mixed model analysis of variance with clusters of varying sizes [10]. Mean changes in other endpoint measures were analyzed for statistical significance by repeated measures analysis of variance.

At baseline, there were no significant differences between the experimental and control groups in demographic characteristics, diet and lifestyle characteristics, functional status, cardiac history, or risk factors. HDL and apolipoprotein A-I were significantly higher in the control group, but ratios of total cholesterol/HDL and LDL/HDL were not significantly different between groups at baseline. At baseline, the experimental and control groups did not significantly differ in disease severity as measured by minimum diameter (D_{min}), percent diameter reduction (%D), normal diameter (D_{norm}), or stenosis flow reserve (SFR).

In the experimental group, adherence to the diet, exercise, and stress management components of the lifestyle program was excellent. Patients in the control group made more moderate changes in lifestyle consistent with more conventional recommendations, including a diet consisting of approximately 30% fat, and 200 mg dietary cholesterol.

In the experimental group, total cholesterol decreased from 226.5 to 171.5 mg/dl (24.3%) and LDL cholesterol fell from 151.4 to 94.8 mg/dl (37.4%). These decreases occurred even though many patients already had made some dietary changes prior to baseline testing. HDL cholesterol did not change significantly in either group. In the experimental group, apolipoprotein B decreased from 104.0 to 78.9, but it did not change appreciably in the control group. Neither group had significant changes in apolipoprotein A-I.

Functional status improved considerably, and in many patients, dramatically. Patients in the experimental group reported a 91% reduction in the frequency of angina, a 42% decrease in duration of angina, and a 28% decrease in the severity of angina. In contrast, control group patients reported a 165% increase in frequency, a 95% increase in duration, and a 39% increase in severity of angina. In our earlier studies, we found that similar improvements in functional status occurred in only one month [1, 2], suggesting that improvements in angina may precede regression of coronary atherosclerosis, perhaps by altering platelet-endothelial interactions, vasomotor tone, or other dynamic characteristics of stenoses.

All detectable lesions were included for analysis. 195 coronary artery lesions were detected and quantitatively analyzed. When all lesions were included, average percent diameter stenosis regressed from 40.0 to 37.8% in the experimental group yet progressed from 42.7 to 46.1% in the control group ($p = 0.001$, two-tailed). When only lesions greater than 50% stenosed were analyzed, average percent diameter stenosis regressed from 61.1 to 55.8% in the experimental group and progressed from 61.7 to 64.4% in the control group ($p = 0.03$, two-tailed).

Eighteen of the 22 patients (82%) in the experimental group had average lesion change scores ($\%D_{post} - \%D_{pre}$) in the direction of regression of coronary atherosclerosis (including the one woman in the experimental group). In contrast, 10 of the 19 control group patients (53%) had average lesion change scores in the direction of progression of coronary atherosclerosis; in contrast, all of the four women in the control group had average lesion change scores in the direction of regression of coronary atherosclerosis.

Within-group secondary analyses were performed to determine if the experimental group showed 'true regression' rather than simply less progression than the control group. In this analysis, the experimental group showed 2.11 ± 0.98 units in the direction of regression ($p = 0.03$, two-tailed). The control group showed 4.23 ± 2.91 units in the direction of progression ($p = 0.15$, two-tailed).

In the experimental group and in the combined groups, overall adherence to the lifestyle changes was strongly related to changes in lesions in a 'dose-response' relationship, suggesting a causal relationship between lifestyle changes and coronary atherosclerosis. These differences in overall adherence are sufficient to explain the observed differences in %D. To assess whether program adherence was related to lesion changes, patients in the experimental group and in the combined groups were divided into three equal tertiles based on overall adherence score. Degree of adherence directly correlated with changes in %D.

This clinical trial demonstrated that a heterogeneous group of patients with coronary heart disease were motivated to make comprehensive changes in lifestyle for at least 1 year in an ambulatory population. These lifestyle changes substantially reduced total cholesterol, LDL cholesterol, and apolipoprotein B, while HDL cholesterol and apolipoprotein A-I remained about the same. These lipid changes are comparable to those seen in studies in which cholesterol-lowering drugs are used. This intervention appears to be safe and compatible with other treatments of coronary heart disease.

After 1 year, patients in the experimental group began to demonstrate significant overall regression of coronary atherosclerosis (decreased %D stenosis) as measured by quantitative coronary arteriography. Since coronary atherosclerosis occurs over a period of decades, one would not expect to find larger changes in only 1 year. Perfusion is a fourth power function of coronary artery diameter, so even a small amount of regression in a critically stenosed artery has a disproportionate effect on myocardial perfusion and thus on functional status and clinical significance.

In contrast, patients in the usual-care control group who were making less comprehensive changes in lifestyle demonstrated significant overall progression of coronary atherosclerosis. This suggests that conventional recommendations for patients with coronary heart disease (such as a 30% fat diet) may not be sufficient to cause regression to occur in many patients, and that more comprehensive lifestyle changes may be required.

The strong relationship between program adherence and lesion changes indicated that most patients needed to follow the lifestyle program as prescribed in order to show regression. Those who made even more changes demonstrated even greater improvement. Since degree of lifestyle change was correlated with degree of stenosis change across the entire range of adherence, even moderate changes in lifestyle may slow the progression of atherosclerosis, whereas substantial changes in lifestyle may be required in order to halt or reverse coronary atherosclerosis.

The five women in the study were the notable exceptions. One woman was randomly assigned to the experimental group and four women were randomly assigned to the control group. All five of these women made only moderate lifestyle changes, yet all showed overall regression. All five were postmenopausal, and none were taking exogenous estrogens. The four women in the control group showed more regression than any of the men in that group, even though some men made greater changes in lifestyle.

While the numbers are small, these data raise the interesting question if gender may influence progression and regression of atherosclerosis.

Five men in the control group also demonstrated very small changes in average %D in the direction of atherosclerosis regression. These patients exercised more often, for longer periods, and consumed fewer calories and less cholesterol than the control group patients who showed progression of atherosclerosis.

The more severely stenosed lesions showed the greatest improvement. Although this is opposite of what was expected, the finding is important since more severely stenotic lesions are of greatest clinical significance. More work is needed to determine to what extent the relationship between change and initial site of lesions is influenced by the statistical phenomenon known as regression to the mean.

Some important questions remain unanswered. Whether or not these comprehensive lifestyle changes can be sustained in larger populations of patients with coronary heart disease remains to be determined. What is optimal is not always easy. Further research will be necessary to determine the mechanisms of changes in coronary atherosclerosis. It would be especially interesting to examine the effects of lifestyle changes in a larger sample of postmenopausal women with coronary atherosclerosis. Also, direct comparisons of intensive lifestyle changes with pharmacologic or surgical interventions are interesting questions needing study. The Lifestyle Heart Trial suggests that comprehensive lifestyle changes may begin to reverse coronary atherosclerosis in only 1 year [11].

If So, What Can Be Done to Achieve Regression of Human Atherosclerosis?

Regression of coronary atherosclerosis in humans has been reported, either in controlled clinical trials or in anecdotal reports, in response to comprehensive lifestyle changes, various cholesterol-lowering drugs, partial ileal bypass surgery, or plasmapheresis. Each of these interventions may be appropriate in some circumstances, either solely or in combination with other interventions. Given these possibilities, what criteria should determine our choice of intervention? The following criteria may be helpful: (1) medical effectiveness; (2) cost-effectiveness; (3) risk-benefit ratio; (4) patient motivation/adherence.

Medical Effectiveness. Comprehensive lifestyle changes may cause significant improvement in risk factors and regression of coronary atherosclerosis. In comparison with other interventions, the Lifestyle Heart Trial measured a greater degree of overall regression in a shorter period of time. However, one should interpret comparisons between studies with caution given the variations from one study to another in patient populations, recruitment, endpoint methodologies, and statistical methods.

Cost-Effectiveness. Cholesterol-lowering medications are costly. Lovastatin, for example, may cost $1,500/year; these costs are considerable when multiplied by the large number of people with hypercholesterolemia. As the goals for desirable plasma cholesterol levels become lower (from 260 to 200 to below 150 mg/dl), the number of people whose plasma cholesterol levels are defined as too high increases. Partial ileal bypass surgery and plasmapheresis are expensive and invasive. In principle, at least, a vegetarian diet, moderate exercise, smoking cessation, and stress management may be learned at moderate cost. While no one has tested this hypothesis, it would not be surprising if comprehensive lifestyle changes may lower utilization of medications (e.g. lipid-lowering drugs) or surgery (e.g. angioplasty or coronary artery bypass surgery), thereby lowering health care costs.

Risk-Benefit Ratio. All drugs, including lipid-lowering medications, have risks and side-effects, both known and unknown, as well as potential benefits. The same is true for plasmapheresis and partial ileal bypass surgery. In contrast, the only side-effects of lifestyle changes are generally desirable ones.

Patient Motivation/Adherence. Clearly, the major obstacle to widespread adoption of comprehensive lifestyle changes is patient adherence. It is often easier to submit to surgery or take medications than to change one's lifestyle. Paradoxically, however, it may be easier to motivate patients to make and maintain comprehensive changes in lifestyle than more moderate ones. When a patient makes only moderate changes in diet and lifestyle, there is often a feeling of deprivation but without substantial improvements in symptoms or plasma cholesterol levels. However, comprehensive lifestyle changes often cause marked reductions in frequency of angina and plasma cholesterol levels, so the choices and benefits become clearer. Patients who, for whatever reason, do not wish to make comprehensive changes in lifestyle should be offered cholesterol-lowering drugs or other options after a clear discussion of the relative risks and benefits of each approach.

In the Lifestyle Heart Trial, we found that adherence to lifestyle changes was strongly correlated with changes in coronary atherosclerosis in a 'dose-response' pattern across the entire range of adherence in both the experimental and control groups. Regression tended to occur when adherence was high even when plasma cholesterol levels did not fall below 150 or even 200 mg/dl. Serum cholesterol levels are important, but coronary heart disease is a multifactorial illness. Evidence suggests that dietary cholesterol and fat may contribute to coronary atherosclerosis in part independent of the effects on plasma cholesterol levels [12, 13]. Algorithms for treating hypercholesterolemia may tend to focus too much on plasma cholesterol levels; attention also should be given to dietary and lifestyle factors.

Is Regression of Human Atherosclerosis Measurable?

Using the methods of quantitative coronary arteriography (QCA) pioneered by Brown et al. [14], Barnt et al. [15], Gould [3], and others, it is now possible to measure the degree of coronary atherosclerosis with reasonable accuracy and reproducibility. This accuracy makes feasible clinical trials with smaller cohorts and shorter durations.

However, coronary arteriography, even when quantitatively analyzed, has some inherent limitations:

(1) Atherosclerosis exists to a considerable degree before it impinges into the arterial lumen. Glagov et al. [16] demonstrated that human coronary arteries undergo compensatory enlargement in the presence of coronary atherosclerosis to preserve the cross-sectional area of the lumen. Coronary arteries enlarge as the lesion area increases, and luminal stenosis may be delayed until the lesion occupies more than 40% of the internal elastic lamina, after which the lumen diminishes markedly. This phenomenon would make it more difficult to detect regression or progression in lesions that are less than 40–50% stenosed at baseline since compensatory changes in the cross-sectional area of the lumen may occur. In contrast, there would be less compensation in more severe lesions, so progression or regression would be easier to measure. Emerging technologies such as intravascular ultrasound may give a more accurate picture of the true extent of coronary atherosclerosis.

(2) It is difficult to distinguish between changes in atherosclerosis and changes in vasomotor tone. If one defines 'regression' as 'clinical improvement', then the question is less important, for both improvements in cor-

onary atherosclerosis and in vasomotor tone increase myocardial perfusion. Giving nitroglycerin at the time of angiography may reduce coronary vasoconstriction; however, this may introduce another confounding variable, for nitroglycerin may not always affect vasomotor tone to the same degree each time in a given patient.

(3) There is no consensus on the best endpoint measure in QCA. Traditionally, percent diameter stenosis (%D) has been used, but there are limitations. %D is a function both of minimum diameter (D_{min}) and the 'normal' segment adjacent to it. However, as discussed by Glagov, even seemingly normal segments are likely to have disease. Also, one may have an apparent improvement in %D if the proximal or distal 'normal' segments narrow and D_{min} is unchanged, since %D is a relative difference between D_{min} and %D. On the other hand, up to a point, a reduction in D_{norm} may paradoxically improve perfusion if D_{min} remains constant due to a reduction in exit losses.

The use of relative percent diameter narrowing as a clinical measure of severity does not account for important other geometric characteristics of stenoses, such as length, absolute cross-sectional luminal area, multiple lesions in series, or eccentric narrowing which may be worse in one view compared to another view. The concept of stenosis flow reserve (SFR) is one way of addressing this dilemma, but it, too, has limitations. The anatomic-geometric approach utilizes all of the X-ray determined geometric dimensions of a stenosis, including percent narrowing, absolute diameter and length effects. These dimensions are integrated throughout the length of the stenosis using fluid dynamic equations to predict the pressure flow characteristics of the stenosis flow reserve (SFR) as a single integrated measure of its severity, reflecting all of the combined effects of percent narrowing, absolute diameter and length. Determination of stenosis flow reserve by this quantitative analysis of coronary arteriograms correlates well with directly measured flow reserve in animals and with perfusion effects in man. In practice, however, SFR is a close function of %D and may not add much additional information. Also, there is little change in SFR until a lesion becomes severely stenosed.

(4) Atherosclerosis is only one of several mechanisms affecting perfusion. Changes in coronary vasomotor tone, platelet adherence and aggregation, collateral circulation, free fatty acid metabolism, local endothelial factors, preload/afterload factors, and other mechanisms may affect myocardial perfusion. Since perfusion is the 'bottom line' in coronary heart disease, functional measures of perfusion (e.g. cardiac PET imaging) may

be a better 'gold standard' than anatomical measures such as coronary arteriography. Both anatomical and functional measures provide complementary information.

(5) 'Not everything that counts can be counted' (Burkitt). We focus on what is measurable, but what is measurable may not necessarily be what is most interesting or important. In the FATS study by Brown et al. [17], for example, there was a 73% reduction in clinical events yet only a 0.7–0.9% diameter stenosis regression in the experimental group.

Thus, mechanisms other than regression of coronary atherosclerosis may play important roles. Psychosocial factors are more difficult to measure, although these, too, may play important roles in both adherence and in outcome [18].

References

1 Ornish DM, Gotto AM, Miller RR, et al: Effects of a vegetarian diet and selected yoga techniques in the treatment of coronary heart disease. Clin Res 1979;27: 720A.
2 Ornish DM, Scherwitz LW, Doody RS, et al: Effects of stress management training and dietary changes in treating ischemic heart disease. JAMA 1983;249:54–59.
3 Gould KL: Identifying and measuring severity of coronary artery stenosis. Quantitative coronary arteriography and positron emission tomography. Circulation 1988; 78:237–245.
4 Stuff JE, Garza C, Smith EO, et al: A comparison of dietary methods in nutritional studies. Am J Clin Nutr 1983;37:300–306.
5 Benson H, Rosner BA, Marzetta BR, Klemchuk HM: Decreased blood pressure in pharmacologically treated hypertensive patients who regularly elicited the relaxation response. Lancet 1974;i:289–291.
6 Ornish D: Reversing Heart Disease. New York, Random House, 1990/Ballantine Books, 1992.
7 Patel C, North WR: Randomised controlled trial of yoga and bio-feedback in management of hypertension. Lancet 1975;ii:93–95.
8 Patel C, Marmot MG, Terry DJ, Carruthers M, Hunt B, Patel M: Trial of relaxation in reducing coronary risk: Four year follow up. Br Med J 1985;290:1103–1106.
9 Orth-Gomer K, Unden AL, Edwards ME: Social isolation and mortality in ischemic heart disease. Acta Med Scand 1988;224:205–215.
10 Dixon WS, et al (eds): BMDP3V Statistical Software; 1983 printing with additions. Berkeley, University of California Press, 1983.
11 Ornish DM, Brown SE, Scherwitz LW, et al: Can lifestyle changes reverse coronary atherosclerosis? The Lifestyle Heart Trial. Lancet 1990;336:129–133.
12 Blankenhorn DH, Johnson RL, El Zein HA, et al: Dietary fat influences human coronary lesion formation. Circulation 1988;78(suppl II):11.

13 Shekelle RB, Stamler J: Dietary cholesterol and ischemic heart disease. Lancet 1989; i:1177–1179.
14 Brown BG, Bolson EL, Dodge HT: Arteriographic assessment of coronary atherosclerosis. Review of current methods, their limitations, and clinical applications. Arteriosclerosis 1982;2:2–15.
15 Barndt R, Blankenhorn DH, Crawford DW, et al: Regression and progression of early femoral atherosclerosis in treated hyperlipoproteinemic patients. Ann Intern Med 1977;86:139–146.
16 Glagov S, Weisenberg E, Zarins CK, et al: Compensatory enlargement of human atherosclerotic coronary arteries. N Engl J Med 1987;316:1371–1375.
17 Brown BG, Alberts JJ, Fisher LD, et al: Regression of coronary artery disease as a result of intensive lipid-lowering therapy in men with high levels of apolipoprotein B. N Engl J Med 1990;323:1289–1298.
18 Ruberman W, Weinblatt E, Goldberg JD, Chaudhary BS: Psychosocial influences on mortality after myocardial infarction. N Engl J Med 1984;311:552–559.

Dean Ornish, MD, Director, Preventive Medicine Research Institute,
University of California, 7 Miller Avenue, Sausalito, CA 94965 (USA)

Simopoulos AP (ed): Nutrition and Fitness in Health and Disease.
World Rev Nutr Diet. Basel, Karger, 1993, vol 72, pp 49–60

Fish and Ischaemic Heart Disease

Michael L. Burr

MRC Epidemiology Unit (South Wales), Llandough Hospital, Penarth, South Glamorgan, UK

Introduction

During recent years interest has arisen in the possibility that dietary fish may confer some protection against ischaemic heart disease (IHD). It was observed that Greenland Eskimos seldom suffered from IHD and had low serum cholesterol and triglyceride concentrations, low platelet aggregability, and a prolonged bleeding time. It seemed reasonable to attribute these characteristics to their diet, which is rich in polyunsaturated fatty acids derived from seafood [1]. Similar associations were reported from studies in Japan [2]. An abrupt change in the Norwegian diet occurred in 1940 and included replacement of meat by fish; within 12 months there was a substantial fall in the incidence and mortality of myocardial infarction (MI) [3].

Fish contain certain long-chain polyunsaturated fatty acids, such as eicosapentaenoic acid (EPA) and docosahexaenoic acid (DHA), which have physiological effects consistent with protection against IHD. These fatty acids are particularly abundant in oily fish such as mackerel, herring, salmon and trout.

Cohort and Case-Control Studies

Table 1 summarizes eight cohort studies of IHD risk in relation to fish intake [4–11]. The Finnish study [4] differed from the others in that it employed stored serum samples rather than dietary data. Four of these studies [4–6, 11] showed a significant inverse association between IHD mortality and fish intake or serum phospholipid EPA concentration; in one [9] there was a non-significant trend; in one [7] there was a non-significant inverse association in a subgroup; and two [8, 10] showed no relationship between IHD and fish intake. The studies with negative or ambivalent findings all lacked a reference group that did not eat fish, however, so that the apparent discrepancy in findings would be explained if protection against IHD is conferred by a fairly low intake. An Italian case-control study supported the inverse relationship between fish and IHD [12]. The fish intake of 287 women with acute MI was significantly lower than that of 649 controls. Two other case-control studies suggested associations between angina and low platelet concentrations of EPA [13, 14].

Clinical Trials

The associations reported in observational studies, such as those considered above, could be attributable to some other characteristic of people who choose to eat fish rather than to the eating of fish per se. More reliable information is supplied by controlled trials in which subjects are randomly

Table 1. Cohort studies of fish and IHD

First author [ref.]	Area	Total subjects	Sex	Group with least fish intake (n)	Associations found
Miettinen [4]	Finland	1,222	M	–	serum EPA inversely with MI and sudden death
Kromhout [5]	Zutphen	852	M	<1 g/day (159)	fish inversely with IHD death
Shekelle [6]	Chicago	1,931	M	<1 g/day (205)	fish inversely with IHD death
Vollset [7]	Norway	11,000	M	0–4 times/month	?fish inversely with IHD death in youngest men only
Curb [8]	Honolulu	7,615	M	'almost never' (32)	none
				none in 24 h	none
Norell [9]	Sweden	10,966	MF	'low consumption'	?fish inversely with IHD death
Lapidus [10]	Gothenburg	1,462	F	none in 24 h	none
Dolecek [11]	USA	6,250	M	none in 4 days ('about 20%')	fish inversely with IHD and all deaths

allocated to receive fish oil or advice to eat more fish. Table 2 presents the results of eight controlled trials of fish oil in preventing restenosis after percutaneous transluminal coronary angioplasty [15–22]. Various other drugs were given to the treatment and control groups, and the duration of treatment prior to angioplasty differed, so that it is difficult to make direct comparisons between these studies. Four [15, 16, 18, 22] showed clear evidence of benefit, in one [17] there was a suggestion of an effect, while in three [19–21] there was no evidence that fish oil was protective. Larger trials are currently in progress which should provide a clearer answer.

A randomized trial in 19 angina patients compared the effects of fish oil and linolenic acid [23]. Both groups of patients improved to a similar extent in respect of symptom frequency and use of glyceryl trinitrate. Another trial compared fish oil with placebo capsules in 8 angina patients, using a randomized double-blind crossover design [24]. There was some improvement in myocardial oxygen demand with fish oil, but no significant changes in symptom frequency, glyceryl trinitrate usage, or exercise tolerance. Both trials were very small, however, and probably had insufficient power to detect any effect likely to occur.

There has been only one randomized trial of fish or fish oil where the outcome was IHD mortality. In this study 2,033 men who had just recovered from MI were randomly allocated to receive various combinations of dietary advice regarding fish, fat, and cereal fibre [25]. A 29% reduction in

Table 2. Randomized controlled trials of fish oil in preventing restenosis after coronary angioplasty

First author [ref.]	Number of subjects followed up	Dose of n–3 fatty acids g/day	Duration months	Assessment	Evidence of benefit
Slack [15]	138	1.8–2.7	6	stress test	yes
Ilsley [16]	108	3.6	6	symptoms, angiography	yes
Milner [17]	149	4.5	6	symptoms, stress, angiography	?yes
Dehmer [18]	82	5.4	6	angiography	yes
Grigg [19]	101	3.0	4	angiography	no
Reis [20]	186	6.0	6	symptoms, angiography	no
Franzen [21]	129	3.15	4	angiography	no
Roy [22]	205	4.5	6	angiography	yes

Table 3. Effects of moderate doses of fish oil on blood lipids

Blood lipid	Type of subject	Effect of fish oil
Cholesterol	normal and hyperlipidaemic	little or no change
Triglyceride	normal and hyperlipidaemic	↓
HDL	normal and hyperlipidaemic	little change in total HDL cholesterol HDL_2 ↑
LDL	normal	?↑
	hyperlipidaemic and diabetic	↑
VLDL	normal and hyperlipidaemic	↓
Chylomicrons	normal	↓

2-year all-cause mortality occurred in the fish advice group in comparison with those not given fish advice. IHD mortality was reduced by 33%, but there was no reduction in non-fatal infarction. The dietary change involved eating about 300 g of fatty fish every week, or taking an equivalent amount of fish oil if the fish could not be tolerated.

Effects on Serum Lipids

Numerous studies have examined the effects of fish oil on blood lipids and lipoproteins; the results are summarized in table 3. Serum cholesterol concentrations are unaffected by doses of fish oil that could be obtained from dietary fish, but serum triglyceride levels are reduced in both normal and hyperlipidaemic subjects, 300 g of fatty fish each week being sufficient to produce this effect [26]. The overall concentration of high-density lipoprotein (HDL) cholesterol is not markedly affected, but a rise in HDL_2 cholesterol (or in the ratio of HDL_2 to HDL_3) has been reported in both normal [27] and hyperlipidaemic [28] subjects. The evidence relating to low density lipoprotein (LDL) cholesterol is less clear. Most studies show little effect of fish oil in healthy subjects, but it has been suggested that a rise occurs if saturated fat intake is kept constant [29]. It also occurs in diabetic patients (both insulin-dependent and non-insulin-dependent) and in several forms of hyperlipidaemia [27]. Very low density lipoprotein (VLDL) concentrations are reduced by fish oil, apparently because both EPA and DHA inhibit the synthesis of VLDL triglyceride [27]. Postpran-

Table 4. Effects of fish oil on certain haemostatic factors

Haemostatic factor	Function	Effect of fish oil
Prostacyclin	prevents platelet aggregation; vasodilatation	PGI_3 ↑
Thromboxane	platelet aggregation; vasoconstriction	TXA_2 ↓
Platelet-activating factor	activates platelets and white cells	↓
Platelet aggregability	blood clotting; plaque formation	↓
Plasma fibrinogen	blood clotting	↓
Blood viscosity	blood clotting	↓
Bleeding time	in vivo test of tendency to bleed	↑

dial lipaemia is reduced and chylomicron clearance is increased if the subjects have been taking fish oil [30], and a dose of 5 g/day seems to be sufficient for this purpose [31].

The changes in serum triglycerides, HDL_2 cholesterol, VLDL and chylomicrons are all consistent with a reduction in the risk of IHD, whereas the rise in LDL cholesterol suggests a possible adverse action.

Effects on Haemostatic Factors

Studies among Eskimos and Japanese drew attention to associations between fish intake, low IHD risk, and a reduced tendency of the blood to clot. These associations have been tested in randomized controlled trials of fish oil, and some of the results are summarized in table 4.

It seems likely that the anti-clotting action of fish oil is mediated largely through the differential production of certain eicosanoids (biologically active 20-carbon molecules derived from arachidonic acid and EPA). Platelet aggregation and arterial tone are controlled by the balance between the eicosanoids prostacyclin (which reduces platelet stickiness and dilates arteries) and thromboxane (which causes platelet aggregation and vasoconstriction). Ingestion of fish oil leads to the replacement of arachidonic acid by EPA in cell membranes, with a consequent modest reduction in the synthesis of the prostacyclin known as prostaglandin I_2 (PGI_2) and an increase in the equally potent PGI_3. There is a corresponding shift from the active thromboxane A_2 (TXA_2) to the relatively inactive TXA_3. The net effect is thus a move in eicosanoid function towards the antithrombotic side [32]. The substitution of EPA and DHA for arachidonic acid also inhibits the formation of platelet-activating factor by monocytes. In consequence of these changes, platelet aggregability markedly declines in persons taking fish oil supplements [33]. Other relevant effects include a reduction in blood viscosity [34] and plasma fibrinogen [35], and a prolongation of the bleeding time [36].

All the above actions are likely to reduce the risk of MI fairly rapidly, and provide an explanation for the observation that an increase in fish intake reduces IHD mortality within about a year [3, 25].

Arterial Effects

Fish oil has a hypotensive effect, both in normotensive [36] and in hypertensive [37] subjects, but the effect is not great and requires more fish oil than would normally be supplied by dietary fish. The mechanisms involved may include a reduction in blood viscosity, reduced TXA_2 production, a reduced response to vasoconstrictors [38], and increased production of PGI_3 and an endothelial-derived relaxing factor [39]. Fish consumption may preserve the compliance of the arterial wall. Aortic compliance was greater in Japanese people living in fishing villages than in those living in farming villages [40]. An Australian study showed that arterial compliance was greater in subjects who ate fish regularly than in those who did not [41].

Several experimental studies have been conducted in animals to see whether fish oil confers protection against atherogenesis. In pigs, fish oil seems to reduce the formation of coronary atheroma induced by diet and balloon abrasion [42, 43], but considerable caution must be exercised in extrapolating the findings to the human disease, which may not behave in the same way as artificially-induced lesions in animals which do not normally eat fish.

Effects on Myocardium

A study in dogs showed that fish oil reduced the size of electrically induced myocardial infarcts and the consequent incidence of ectopic beats [44]. In rats, fish oil reduces ischaemic damage following coronary ligation

[45]; it also prevents ventricular fibrillation induced by stress [46], by acute ischaemia, or by reperfusion following ischaemia [47]. In the marmoset monkey (a species whose blood lipid profile and myocardial innervation resemble those of man) fish oil improves cardiac function and prevents ventricular fibrillation occurring upon electrical stimulation or coronary artery ligation [48]. EPA solution protects rat cardiac myocytes in vitro from the arrhythmogenic toxic effects of ouabain [49]. It is possible that the action of fish oil on risk of arrhythmia is mediated by a change in the balance of myocardial eicosanoids since TXA_2 seems to be arrhythmogenic and PGI_2 anti-arrhythmogenic [48].

One randomized controlled trial found no anti-arrhythmogenic effect of fish oil in man [50]. But this trial contained only 18 subjects, and their frequency of arrhythmia was initially low. This trial does not therefore provide strong evidence against an anti-arrhythmic action. A case-control study showed that men who suffered sudden cardiac death had a higher ratio of arachidonic acid to DHA in cardiac phospholipids than men who died suddenly in accidents [46].

It would obviously be unwise to conclude from animal and in vitro studies that fish oil limits ischaemic damage or prevents arrhythmia in man. But the experimental evidence at least suggests these possibilities, which would explain the fact that fish seemed to prevent death but not reinfarction in men recovering from MI [25].

Fish or Fish Oil?

Are dietary fish and fish oil supplements equally effective in preventing heart disease? Population and cohort studies are necessarily based on the eating of fish, since this is what people do spontaneously. Experimental studies, on the other hand, usually employ fish oil capsules, since their dosage can be controlled more precisely, the diet is unaffected, and trials can be double-blind with the use of matching placebo capsules. The one trial showing an effect on mortality was based mostly on dietary fish but with some fish oil supplementation, and it was not possible to analyze these groups separately as relatively few subjects took fish oil.

There are substantial reasons for believing that the protective effects of dietary fish are attributable to the long-chain fatty acids of the omega–3 series, particularly EPA and DHA, which characterize fish oil. Dietary fish and fish oil produce similar changes in blood lipids and haemostatic fac-

Table 5. IHD mortality in MRFIT usual care participants, according to sum of dietary 20:5, 22:5 and 22:6 omega–3 fatty acids [11]

Daily omega–3 intake		Total	IHD deaths		Relative risks (adjusted*)
quintile	mean, g		n	%	
I	0.000	1,307	42	3.21	1.00
II	0.009	1,197	39	3.26	1.08
III	0.046	1,251	35	2.80	0.91
IV	0.153	1,252	35	2.80	0.88
V	0.664	1,251	24	1.92	0.60

* Adjusted for age and other baseline risk factors.

Table 6. Mortality and IHD events in men who had recently recovered from MI, according to EPA intake

EPA intake g/week	Total	Mean age at entry years	Deaths		IHD events	
			n	%	n	%
<1	114	56.1	7	6.1	9	7.9
1–2	373	57.0	19	5.1	26	7.0
≥2	460	56.3	19	4.1	31	6.7

Unpublished data from Diet and Reinfarction Trial [25].

tors, and these changes are consistent with a reduction in risk of IHD. The one cohort study which examined intake of specific fatty acids [11] found an inverse dose-response relationship between long-chain omega–3 fatty acids and IHD mortality (table 5). Data [hitherto unpubl.] from the secondary prevention trial of fatty fish [25] similarly suggest a dose-response effect of omega–3 fatty acids: the EPA intakes at 6 months in the fish advice group were inversely related to mortality and IHD events during the following 18 months (table 6). Although this relationship might be just a 'healthy complier' effect (the same trend was seen with regard to cereal fibre, which conferred no benefit overall), it is at least consistent with a protective action of omega–3 fatty acids. There are of course many other ingredients of fish, but there is no evidence that they have relevant effects of comparable importance.

It therefore seems exceedingly likely that fish prevents heart disease by means of its long-chain fatty acids. The question then arises as to the most efficient method of their administration: fish or fish oil.

One study compared the effects of fish and fish oil supplying equal amounts of EPA plus DHA. Plasma concentrations of triglycerides and VLDL triglyceride fell and HDL_2 cholesterol rose equally in the two groups, but only the fish affected the haemostatic factors (reducing fibrinogen and thromboxane and prolonging the bleeding time) [51], possibly because of its higher DHA content. The relative proportions of these fatty acids may thus be important. Furthermore, EPA may be absorbed more efficiently from fish than from fish oil [52]. It may be possible to obtain benefit equally from fatty fish and fish oil, if sufficient capsules are taken. But for most people the fish will be preferred as far more palatable and enjoyable than the capsules.

Conclusions

People who eat fish are less likely to die of IHD than people who do not. One randomized controlled trial suggests that fatty fish reduces the risk of death in men who have recently recovered from MI. The protective mechanism is uncertain, but it may involve a reduced tendency of blood to clot, or a reduction in ventricular arrhythmias, and appears to be attributable to the long-chain omega–3 fatty acids which characterize oily fish.

References

1 Dyerberg J, Bang HO: Haemostatic function and platelet polyunsaturated fatty acids in Eskimos. Lancet 1979;ii:433–435.
2 Hirai A, Terano T, Tamura Y, et al: Eicosapentaenoic acid and adult disease in Japan: Epidemiological and clinical aspects. J Intern Med 1989;225(suppl 1): 69–75.
3 Bang HO, Dyerberg J: Personal reflections on the incidence of ischaemic heart disease in Oslo during the Second World War. Acta Med Scand 1981;210:245–248.
4 Miettinen TA, Naukkarinen V, Hattunen JK, et al: Fatty-acid composition of serum lipids predicts myocardial infarction. Br Med J 1982;285:993–996.

5 Kromhout D, Bosschieter EB, Coulander CdeL: The inverse relation between fish consumption and 20-year mortality from coronary heart disease. N Engl J Med 1985;312:1205–1209.
6 Shekelle RB, Missell L, Paul O, et al: Fish consumption and mortality from coronary heart disease. N Engl J Med 1985;313:820.
7 Vollset S, Heuch I, Bjelke E: Fish consumption and mortality from coronary heart disease. N Engl J Med 1985;313:820–821.
8 Curb JD, Reed DM: Fish consumption and mortality from coronary heart disease. N Engl J Med 1985;313:821.
9 Norell SE, Ahlbom A, Feychting M, et al: Fish consumption and mortality from coronary heart disease. Br Med J 1986;293:426.
10 Lapidus L, Andersson H, Bengtsson C, et al: Dietary habits in relation to incidence of cardiovascular disease and death in women: A 12-year follow-up of participants in the population study of women in Gothenburg, Sweden. Am J Clin Nutr 1986;44: 444–448.
11 Dolecek TA, Grandits G: Dietary polyunsaturated fatty acids and mortality in the multiple risk factor intervention trial (MRFIT). World Rev Nutr Diet 1991;66:205–216.
12 Gramenzi A, Gentile A, Fasoli M, et al: Association between certain foods and risk of acute myocardial infarction in women. Br Med J 1990;300:771–773.
13 Prisco D, Rogasi PG, Matucci M, et al: Increased thromboxane A2 generation and altered membrane fatty acid composition in platelets from patients with active angina pectoris. Thromb Res 1986;44:101–112.
14 Wood DA, Riemersma RA, Butler S, et al: Linoleic and eicosapentaenoic acids in adipose tissue and platelets and risk of coronary heart disease. Lancet 1987;i:177–183.
15 Slack JD, Pinkerton CA, Van Tassel J, et al: Can oral fish oil supplement minimize restenosis after percutaneous transluminal coronary angioplasty? J Am Coll Cardiol 1987;9:64A.
16 Ilsley CDJ, Nye ER, Sutherland W, et al: Randomised placebo-controlled trial of maxepa and aspirin/persantin after successful coronary angioplasty. Aust NZ J Med 1987;17:559.
17 Milner MR, Gallino RA, Leffingwell A, et al: High dose omega-3 fatty acid supplementation reduces clinical restenosis after coronary angioplasty. Circulation 1988; 78(suppl II):634.
18 Dehmer GJ, Popma JJ, van den Berg EK, et al: Reduction in the rate of early restenosis after coronary angioplasty by a diet supplemented with n-3 fatty acids. N Engl J Med 1988;319:733–740.
19 Grigg LE, Kay TWH, Valentine PA, et al: Determinants of restenosis and lack of effect of dietary supplementation with eicosapentaenoic acid on the incidence of coronary artery restenosis after angioplasty. J Am Coll Cardiol 1989;13:665–672.
20 Reis GJ, Boucher TM, Sipperly ME, et al: Randomised trial of fish oil for prevention of restenosis after coronary angioplasty. Lancet 1989;ii:177–181.
21 Franzen D, Höpp HW, Günther H, et al: Prospective, randomized and double-blinded trial about the effect of fish oil on the incidence of restenosis following PTCA and on coronary artery disease progression. Eur Heart J 1990;11(abstr suppl): 367.

22 Roy L, Bairati I, Meyer F, et al: Double-blind randomized controlled trial of fish oil supplements in the prevention of restenoses after coronary angioplasty. Circulation 1991;84(suppl II):365.
23 Kristensen SD, Schmidt EB, Andersen HR, et al: Fish oil in angina pectoris. Atherosclerosis 1987;64:13–19.
24 Mehta JL, Lopez LM, Lawson D, et al: Dietary supplementation with omega-3 polyunsaturated fatty acids in patients with stable coronary heart disease: Effects on indices of platelet and neutrophil function and exercise performance. Am J Med 1988;84:45–52.
25 Burr ML, Fehily AM, Gilbert JF, et al: Effects of changes in fat, fish and fibre intakes on death and myocardial reinfarction: diet and reinfarction trial (DART). Lancet 1989;ii:757–761.
26 Fehily AM, Burr ML, Phillips KM, et al: The effect of fatty fish on plasma lipid and lipoprotein concentrations. Am J Clin Nutr 1983;38:349–351.
27 Sanders TAB: Influence of ω3 fatty acids on blood lipids. World Rev Nutr Diet 1991;66:358–366.
28 Abbey M, Clifton P, Kestin M, et al: Effect of fish oil on lipoproteins, lecithin: cholesterol acyltransferase, and lipid transfer protein activity in humans. Arteriosclerosis 1990;10:85–94.
29 Fumeron F, Brigant L, Ollivier V, et al: n–3 polyunsaturated fatty acids raise low-density lipoproteins, high-density lipoprotein 2, and plasminogen-activator inhibitor in healthy young men. Am J Clin Nutr 1991;54:118–122.
30 Weintraub MS, Zechner R, Brown A, et al: Dietary polyunsaturated fats of the W–6 and W–3 series reduce postprandial lipoprotein levels. Chronic and acute effects of fat saturation on postprandial lipoprotein metabolism. J Clin Invest 1988;82:1884–1893.
31 Brown AJ, Roberts DCK: Moderate fish oil intake improves lipemic response to a standard fat meal. A study in 25 healthy men. Arterioscler Thromb 1991;11:457–466.
32 Weber PC, Leaf A: Cardiovascular effects of ω3 fatty acids. World Rev Nutr Diet 1991;66:218–232.
33 Brox JH, Killie J-E, Gunnes S, et al: The effect of cod liver oil and corn oil on platelets and vessel wall in man. Thromb Haemostas 1981;46:604–611.
34 Woodcock BE, Smith E, Lambert WH, et al: Beneficial effect of fish oil on blood viscosity in peripheral vascular disease. Br Med J 1984;288:592–594.
35 Hostmark AT, Bjerkedal T, Kierulf P, et al: Fish oil and plasma fibrinogen. Br Med J 1988;297:180–181.
36 Mortensen JZ, Schmidt EB, Nielsen AH, et al: The effect of N–6 and N–3 polyunsaturated fatty acids on hemostasis, blood lipids and blood pressure. Thromb Haemostas 1983;50:543–546.
37 Knapp HR, Fitzgerald GA: The antihypertensive effects of fish oil: A controlled study of polyunsaturated fatty acid supplements in essential hypertension. N Engl J Med 1989;320:1037–1043.
38 Lorenz R, Spengler U, Fischer S, et al: Platelet function, thromboxane formation and blood pressure control during supplementation of the Western diet with cod liver oil. Circulation 1983;67:504–511.

39 Shimokawa H, Lam JYT, Chesebro JH, et al: Effects of dietary supplementation with cod-liver oil on endothelium-dependent responses in porcine coronary arteries. Circulation 1987;76:898–905.
40 Hamazake T, UrakazeM, Sawazaki S, et al: Comparison of pulse wave velocity of the aorta between inhabitants of fishing and farming villages in Japan. Atherosclerosis 1988;73:157–160.
41 Wahlqvist ML, Lo CS, Myers KA: Fish intake and arterial wall characteristics in healthy people and diabetic patients. Lancet 1989;ii:944–946.
42 Weiner BH, Ockene IS, Levine PH, et al: Inhibition of atherosclerosis by cod-liver oil in a hyperlipidemic swine model. N Engl J Med 1986;315:841–846.
43 Sassen LMA, Hartog JM, Lamers JMJ, et al: Mackerel oil and atherosclerosis in pigs. Eur Heart J 1989;10:838–:846.
44 Culp BR, Lands WEM, Lucchesi BR, et al: The effect of dietary supplementation of fish oil on experimental myocardial infarction. Prostaglandins 1980;20:1021–1031.
45 Hock CE, Holahan MA, Reibel DK: Effect of dietary fish oil on myocardial phospholipids and myocardial ischemic damage. Am J Physiol 1987;252:H554–H560.
46 Gudbjarnason S: Dynamics of n–3 and n–6 fatty acids in phospholipids of heart muscle. J Int Med 1989;225(suppl 1):117–128.
47 McLennan PL, Abeywardena MY, Charnock JS: Reversal of the arrhythmogenic effects of long-term saturated fatty acid intake by dietary n–3 and n–6 polyunsaturated fatty acids. Am J Clin Nutr 1990;51:53–58.
48 Charnock JS: Antiarrhythmic effects of fish oils. World Rev Nutr Diet 1991;66: 278–291.
49 Hallaq H, Sellmayer A, Smith TW, et al: Protective effect of eicosapentaenoic acid on ouabain toxicity in neonatal rat cardiac myocytes. Proc Natl Acad Sci USA 1990; 87:7834–7838.
50 Hardarson T, Kristinsson A, Skuladottir G, et al: Cod liver oil does not reduce ventricular extrasystoles after myocardial infarction. J Int Med 1989;226:33–37.
51 Cobiac L, Clifton PM, Abbey M, et al: Lipid, lipoprotein, and hemostatic effects of fish vs fish-oil n–3 fatty acids in mildly hyperlipidemic males. Am J Clin Nutr 1991; 53:1210–1216.
52 Silverman DI, Ware JA, Sacks FM, et al: Comparison of the absorption and effect on platelet function of a single dose of n–3 fatty acids given as fish or fish oil. Am J Clin Nutr 1991;53:1165–1170.

Michael L. Burr, MD, University of Wales College of Medicine,
Temple of Peace and Health, Cathays Park, Cardiff CF1 3NW (UK)

Simopoulos AP (ed): Nutrition and Fitness in Health and Disease.
World Rev Nutr Diet. Basel, Karger, 1993, vol 72, pp 61–67

Implementation and Mobilization of Resources

Alexander Leaf

Harvard Medical School, Massachusetts General Hospital, Boston, Mass., and Department of Veterans Affairs Medical Center, Brockton/West Roxbury, Mass., USA

At each Olympic Games new world records are set as successive generations of athletes out-perform their predecessors. Superior coaching and more intensive training are rightly credited for the progressive improvements in athletic performance. Often another important factor is overlooked. The pool of athletes from which the Olympic competitors are drawn has been gradually expanding over the centuries and increasingly so in the past few decades. As the popularity of sports has spread from a few countries to many, the number of competitive athletes has increased as well. Modern communications have done much to spread the addiction to athletic competition around the world so that with each Olympic Games the number of participating countries increases. Despite the broad geographic representation at the Games, however, the proportion of young people in most countries capable of attaining the level of physical performance required for competitive athletics is very small. Genetic limitations in neuro-musculo-skeletal, cardiovascular or pulmonary endowment account for some of this host of unfit young adults. The great majority of this unfit host, however, results from unfortunate circumstances – poor nutrition, disease, habits of slothfulness and lack of education.

Paradoxically, the nutritional-based dysfunction results from both excesses and deficiencies. I would like to discuss each, the circumstances under which they occur, and remedies that are urgently needed for their correction.

Primarily in affluent, Western industrialized countries an abundance of readily available, high caloric, fatty, and nutritionally empty foods have contributed to the epidemic of obesity and coronary heart disease which afflicts these countries. Emergence of affluent segments of societies even in the developing world has extended the health problem to global dimensions. Although these cultures provide the majority of competitive athletes, their numbers are dwarfed by their physically unfit compatriots. It is now well established that the arterial changes which result in later heart attacks are already manifest in adolescence and early adulthood. Though the arterial lesions at this stage are unlikely to limit physical performance, the associated obesity, hypertension, cigarette smoking and – all too often – alcohol and drug abuse, surely will. In the midst of affluence and abundance, life-style choices become paramount in determining health and physical fitness.

Our children need to be indoctrinated at an early age in habits of good nutrition for optimal health. This includes proper nutrition of all expectant mothers and universal breast feeding of all infants to give each child the best start in life. Eating habits of the family should provide a diet low in saturated fat with ample levels of omega-6 and omega-3 polyunsaturated fatty acids, a diversity of fresh vegetables, legumes, fruits, and grains. Fats should comprise no more than 20–25% of calories; protein from lean meats, poultry, fish, and dairy products should add another 10–15% of calories; and the remainder should be provided by unrefined carbohydrates. Such diets should be adequate in vitamins, trace elements and all nutrients, and be free of infectious and toxic contaminants. This is not the place to provide details of specific menus to provide the requisite nutrition, but these overall guidelines should support optimal growth and health for future athletes and productive citizens. Eating habits that begin in the family need to be reinforced in elementary and secondary schools with instruction that provides at least an informed explanation why such diets are essential for optimal performance of our bodies at all stages of life. Every effort should be made to reduce temptations to smoke, consume alcohol, abuse drugs, and engage in early and unhealthy sexual practices. The great majority of such self-destructive habits are acquired before the age of 18–20 years and are antithetical to optimal health and fitness. Very important in this regard is the need to challenge our youth with educational, vocational and career opportunities to develop their sense of self-esteem and engage their participation in socially beneficial activities in democratic and free societies.

Obviously, essential for optimal fitness is a program of physical exercise which will be practiced on a regular daily basis throughout life. The healthy exuberance and vitality of young children is expressed naturally in physical activity. This needs to be encouraged in the older child and adolescent by physical education courses in primary and secondary schools which, in addition to providing time for exercises and participation in sports, should educate each student to the benefits to general health of aerobic, endurance exercises. Students should be encouraged to develop habits of regular aerobic endurance exercises which they can enjoy throughout life. Walking, jogging, cycling, swimming, rowing, cross-country skiing are the models of such exercises which can be performed in many forms daily or at least three times weekly to develop and sustain fitness. With all youth and young adults engaged in such regular exercises, general performance in sports must improve and the number of gifted athletes arising from such a large, physically fit, healthy cohort will assure continued setting of world records in future Olympic competitions.

Sadly, the other aspect of the nutritional and health paradox mentioned, represents a much larger destruction and wastage of human resources than the sins of affluence, just discussed. The United Nations Children's Fund (UNICEF) opens its remarkable treatise *The State of the World's Children 1992* [1] with the bald statement: 'A quarter of a million of the world's young children are dying every week, and millions more are surviving in the half-life of malnutrition and almost permanent ill health.' These are the children who are the victims of preventable malnutrition, disease, and illiteracy. They are being most shamefully failed by the present world order. This shameful situation demands correction, not only for moral and ethical reasons and for the enormous waste in human potential it entails, but even more immediately for the economic and environmental disaster we are creating in our world by pursuing policies that create such human disaster.

This situation was the central theme of the *World Summit for Children* in September, 1990 which brought together for 2 days leaders from over 150 nations including 71 Presidents and Prime Ministers. The Summit Declaration [2] set some 27 goals to be attained by the year 2000. These goals include a one-third reduction in child deaths, a halving of child malnutrition, a halving of deaths among women during pregnancy and childbirth, universally available family planning, safe water and sanitation for all, and basic education for all children. More specifically the goals include 90% immunization, polio eradication, the elimination of neonatal tetanus, a 95% reduction in measles deaths (currently about 840,000 annually), a halving of child deaths caused by diarrhea (4 million a year) and a one-third reduction in child deaths from pneumonia (3 million a year).

At first sight tackling so many goals at once may seem overly ambitious, but as *The State of the World's Children 1992* [1] indicates, a close inter-relation between the goals makes this feasible. Reducing child malnutrition, for example, sharply reduces child deaths. Reduced child deaths means that more parents become interested in family planning. More family planning improves maternal and child health, leading in turn to better nutrition and fewer deaths, but also to reduction in population growth and the opportunity to reduce global environmental pollution. The know-how and the technology to attain these goals is available. The network for accomplishing the immunization goals has been established. The total cost to attain these goals was estimated at $20 billion a year throughout the 1990s and at least one-third of this would need to come from increases in, or a reallocation of, international aid [1]. The extra aid required is estimated to amount to less than 1% of the industrialized world's current military expenditures. In the post cold war era, this would hardly seem too high a price to pay to save the lives of many millions of children, prevent the malnutrition of many millions more, slow the world's rate of population growth, and make perhaps the greatest of all investments in the future.

This is not the appropriate place to discuss the details of what needs to be done to realize the goals of the *World Summit for Children. The State of the World's Children 1992* has laid out ten propositions aimed to achieve the goals and these are ennumerated in table 1 [1].

I do not mean to leave the impression that these measures are needed only in the developing countries in the world. In the United States, for example, the proportion of children living in poverty has risen from 14% in the 1960s to approximately 22% today [3]! Exploding the myth that this is attributable solely to an increase in inner-city blacks and Hispanics, the *Children's Defense Fund* indicates that the majority of the United States' 12 million poor children are white; most live outside big cities; most live in families with only one or two children; and most belong to households where at least one parent works [3]. Sadly we must realize that poverty is taking its toll on children the world over.

A particularly onerous situation has been created over the past decade. More than one and a half million children have been killed in wars [4], more than 4 million have been disabled – limbs amputated, brains damaged, eyesight and hearing lost – through bombing, land-mines, firearms, and torture. Five million children are in refugee camps because of war and a further 12 million have lost their homes. This 'war on children' is a 20th

Table 1. The ten propositions of the State of the World's Children [1]

1	That the promise of the World Summit for Children should be kept and that a new world order should bring an end to malnutrition, preventable disease, and illiteracy among so many millions of the world's children.
2	That the principle of 'first call for children' – meaning that protection for the growing bodies and minds of the young ought to have a first call on societies' resources – should become an accepted ethic of a new world order.
3	That if the issues of malnutrition, preventable disease, and widespread illiteracy, are not confronted as a new world order evolves, then it will be very much more difficult to reduce the rate of population growth and make the transition to environmentally sustainable development.
4	That the growing consensus around the importance of market economic policies should be accompanied by a corresponding consensus on the responsibility of governments to guarantee basic investments in people.
5	That increases in international aid should be based on a sustained and measurable commitment to meeting minimum human needs and for maintaining, in difficult times, the principle of a first call for children.
6	That international action on debt, aid, and trade should create an environment in which economic reform in the developing world can succeed in allowing its people to earn a decent living.
7	That a process of demilitarization should begin in the developing world and that, in step with that process, falling military expenditures in the industrialized nations should be linked to significant increases in international aid for development and for the resolution of common global problems.
8	That the chains of Africa's debt be struck off and that the continent be given sufficient external support to allow internal reform to succeed in regenerating the momentum of development.
9	That a new world order should oppose the apartheid of gender as vigorously as the apartheid of race.
10	That the responsible planning of births is one of the most effective and least expensive ways of improving the quality of life on earth – both now and in the future – and that one of the greatest mistakes of our times is the failure to realise that potential.

century invention. Only 5% of casualties in the First World War were civilians. By the Second World War, the proportion had risen to 50%. As the century ends, the civilian share is normally about 80% – mostly women and children. This results from what we are told are 'surgically clean wars', which destroy facilities and resources, but not people.

Since most of us here are health professionals, I will conclude this conscience-raising message with only one further discomforting health statistic. World-wide we are spending many times more money on 'curative' than on preventive health measures. For 75% of public spending on health to serve only the richest 25% of the population, is not atypical [5]; for more to be spent on sophisticated operations than on the low-cost control of mass disease, is not uncommon [6]; for 30% of the health budgets of some poor countries to be spent on sending a privileged few for treatments abroad, is not unknown [7].

It seems urgent that we act in concert to implement the promise of *The World Summit for Children.* If a new World Order is to have meaning in our time, such action is essential. All aspects of life on our planet should benefit from achieving the stated goals.

Conclusions and Recommendations

(1) All countries should join forces to implement the goals of the *World Summit for Children* as stated in the *Summit Declaration* [2], so that all children can start life with a potential for fitness based on optimal health.

(2) All children should receive a healthful, nutritious diet without excesses or deficiencies of calories or essential nutrients.

(3) All children should have the opportunity to engage in physical fitness programs which emphasize the importance of aerobic, endurance type physical activities and to receive instruction in school of the health benefits of such exercise. Adoption of pleasurable forms of activity that can be enjoyed throughout life on a regular and frequent basis, should be encouraged.

(4) All children should be helped to avoid use of tobacco, abuse of drugs and alcohol and to abstain from early, unhealthy sexual practices.

(5) A positive self-image for all children should be fostered by universal access to education, and fulfilling career opportunities.

(6) Universal access to health care for all children should be provided with emphasis on primary care and preventive medicine. The goal of such health care should be to prevent illness and optimize health for as long as the individual's biological life span permits. Promotion of good nutrition and regular aerobic physical exercise for all throughout life must be mainstays of such a health care system.

References

1 Grant JP: The State of the World's Children 1992. London, Oxford University Press, 1991.
2 Summit Declaration and Plan of Action and Convention on the Rights of the Child: The State of the World's Children 1991. London, Oxford University Press, 1991.
3 Johnson CM, Miranda L, Sherman A, Weill JD: Child Poverty in America. Children's Defense Fund, 122 C Street, N.W., Washington, DC 20001, 1991.
4 Effects of Armed Conflict on Women and Children: Relief and Rehabilitation in War Situations, vol 10, issue 2–3, 1991. Rehabilitation International and UNICEF, Technical Support Programme for the United Nations Decade of Disabled Persons (1983–1992).
5 Cornia GA: Child Poverty and Deprivation in Industrialized Countries: Recent Trends and Policy Options. Florence, UNICEF, International Child Development Centre, Innocenti Occasional Papers No 2, 1990, pp 175–176.
6 World Bank: World Development Report 1991. Washington, World Bank, 1991, p 66.
7 Nakajima H: Interview with the Director-General, World Health Organization; in Development Forum, vol xviii, No 2. New York, United Nations Department of Public Information, 1990.

Alexander Leaf, MD, Massachusetts General Hospital, East, 4th Floor,
Building 149, 13th Street, Charlestown, MA 02129 (USA)

Panel IV
Obesity

Simopoulos AP (ed): Nutrition and Fitness in Health and Disease.
World Rev Nutr Diet. Basel, Karger, 1993, vol 72, pp 68–77

Genetics of Obesity and Its Prevention

Claude Bouchard

Physical Activity Sciences Laboratory, Laval University, Ste-Foy, Qué., Canada

Energy balance is commonly defined as the result of prevailing energy intake and energy expenditure conditions. If energy intake and total energy expenditure are not equal for a given period of time, a change in body energy content will necessarily occur. The focus of this short review is on individual differences in body energy content and in major affectors of body energy content. For practical reasons, body fat content or body mass for stature are generally used to classify patients on a scale that may typically include the following categories: underweight, normal or healthy weight, overweight, obese or severely obese. One can argue, however, that body energy content relative to stature or stature squared would be a more appropriate phenotype [1]. Body energy content is a phenotype resulting from a complex network of genetic and nongenetic influences. Such phenotypes are known as multifactorial phenotypes.

A Model of the Major Affectors

Individual differences are determined by variations in energy balance, a positive energy balance over a relatively long period of time resulting in an increase in the phenotype. However, we still do not have a clear understanding of all the complex mechanisms coupling energy intake and energy expenditure. We understand that both are generally not highly coupled over a short period of time but are reasonably well correlated in the long run in the normal weight individuals. In some cases, apparently high levels of energy intake in sedentary persons do not appear to be accompanied by positive energy balance. In others, low levels of dietary energy while the individuals remain sedentary translate into positive energy balance and weight gain.

A high level of habitual physical activity generally translates into a low body energy content. Adipose tissue lipoprotein lipase activity is often quite high in those with a high body energy content for stature (e.g. the obese or even the reduced obese). However, at this time, it is not clear whether it is a cause or an effect of the condition. Composition of the diet, resting metabolic rate, thermic response to food, proportion of lipid oxidized, and proneness to store energy in the form of fat or lean tissue are of particular interest. A high fat diet is becoming increasingly recognized as a factor that enhances the risk of being in positive energy balance. The resting metabolic rate is weakly correlated with weight gain over time, thus with positive energy balance. A depressed thermic response to food is observed in a subgroup of obese individuals but not in all of them. The respiratory exchange ratio, an estimate of the relative proportion of lipid and carbohydrate oxidized, is also weakly correlated with weight gain over time. Finally, the proneness to store excess food energy as fat or lean tissue is a correlate of body energy content.

Figure 1 presents a summary of the major classes of affectors of body energy content for stature. The interactions between the various classes of affectors are also illustrated. For a given individual, these affectors, if they could all be assessed successfully, would likely specify energy balance provided energy losses in the feces and urine were taken into account [2].

In brief, energy intake includes not only the total caloric intake, but also the macronutrient composition of the intake, the palatability of the diet, its content of various amino acids and other molecules as they influence the metabolic outcomes of the food ingested, and appetite as well as satiety. Energy expenditures include basal and resting metabolic rates, thermic effect of food, energy cost of exercise and work, level of habitual physical activity, temperature-induced thermogenesis, stress-induced thermogenesis and other components.

The next component is probably the most complex. It is defined as the interface between energy or nutrient intake and expenditure and results from the fact that there are characteristics of the human body that have an impact on the outcome of a given set of energy intake and expenditure conditions. Variations in the biological/behavioral interface can be caused by inherited or acquired conditions. For instance, one could find inherited

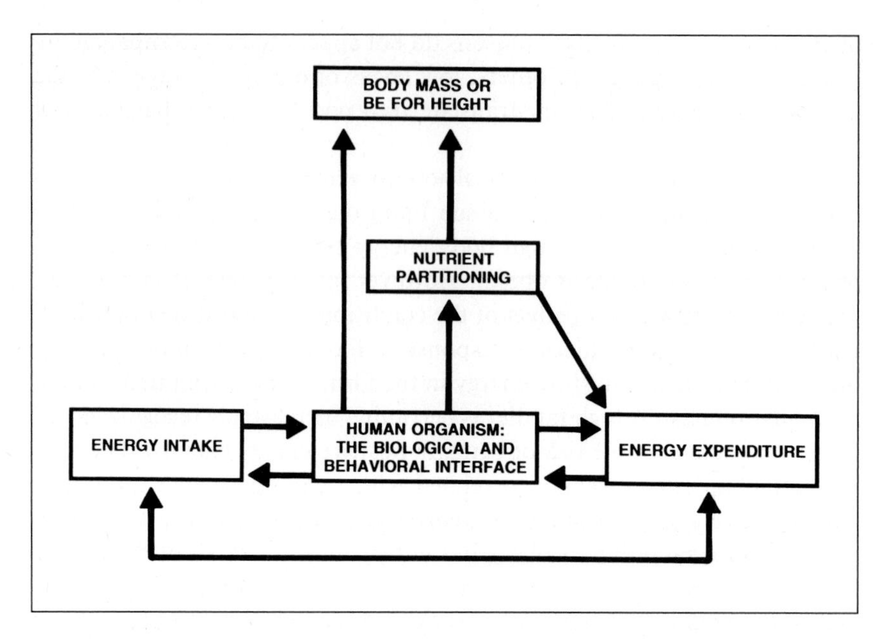

Fig. 1. A paradigm of the major affectors of body energy (BE) content or body mass for stature.

variants in enzymes of the liver (or other tissues) that may influence the efficiency of lipid metabolism in the carrier individuals and effect substrate utilization under certain dietary conditions. This in turn may impact on energy balance and influence body energy content. Finally, a critical determinant of total body energy content for stature is nutrient partitioning. Indeed, the proneness to store ingested energy relatively more or less in the form of triacylglycerides in adipose tissue or as lean tissue is an important factor.

Heritability of Body Energy Content

During the last 60 years or so, a large number of authors have reported that obese parents had a higher risk of having obese children than lean parents. This does not constitute a clear demonstration that the obesity of the offspring is determined by the so-called 'obesity' genes of the parents as both generations share not only genes but also the household milieu and many environmental conditions. Nonetheless, they clearly suggest that having an obese mother or one obese parent meant a greater risk of becoming obese [3].

Based on a stratified sample of the Canadian population, several skinfolds were available on about 18,000 subjects living in more than 10,000 different households [4]. We were able to establish that the total transmission effect across generations for the age and gender adjusted sum of 5 skinfolds reached about 35%. We have also reported on the genetic effect in fat mass and percent body fat measured with one of the commonly accepted direct methods for measuring body composition [5]. In this research, we had performed underwater weighing measurements of body density in a relatively large number of individuals belonging to 9 different kinds of relatives. About half of the variance, after adjustment for age and gender, in fat mass or percent body fat was associated with a transmissible effect and 25% of the variance was an additive genetic effect. Using the same database, the additive genetic effect for body energy content adjusted for age, gender and height reached only 15% [6]. One must keep in mind that the study was conducted on a sample with only a small number of obese subjects. In the same study based largely on normal weight and moderately overweight subjects, no specific maternal or paternal effects as well as no sex-limited effects could be detected for subcutaneous fat or total body fat [5]. The genetic epidemiology of body energy content or obesity based on large samples of lean and obese subjects, with valid assessment procedures, is a task for the future.

Response to Overfeeding

It is generally recognized that there are some individuals prone to excessive accumulation of fat, for which losing weight represents a continuous battle, and others who seem relatively well protected against such a menace. We have attempted to test whether such differences could be accounted for by inherited differences. In other words, we asked whether there were differences when chronically exposed to positive energy balance and whether such differences were dependent or independent of the genotype. If the answer to both questions was affirmative then one would have to conclude that there was a significant genotype-environment interaction effect.

Twelve pairs of male identical twins were subjected to a 4.2 MJ per day caloric surplus, 6 days a week, during a period of 100 days for a total overfeeding stimulus of 353 MJ [7]. Significant increases in body weight, fat mass, fat free mass, and body energy content were observed after the period of overfeeding. Data showed that there were considerable interindividual differences in the adaptation to excess calories and that the variation observed was not randomly distributed, as indicated by the significant within pair resemblance in response. There was at least 3 times more variance in response between pairs than within pairs for the gains in body mass, fat mass, fat free mass and body energy content. These data demonstrate that some individuals are more at risk than others to gain fat when energy intake surplus is clamped at the same level for everyone and when subjects are confined to a sedentary lifestyle. The within identical twin pair response to the standardized caloric surplus suggests that the amount of body energy gained is likely influenced by the genotype. The genetic effect is, however, moderate and accounts for only about 50% of the variation in the response to the overfeeding protocol.

Food Preference

Familial resemblance in nutrient intake has been reported in spouses as well as in parents and their children. Results from twin studies showed that monozygotic twins were more alike than dizygotic twins regarding their diets [8, 9]. Moreover, a genetic influence on the concentration of nutrients in the diet [8] and on the selection of some foods [10], particularly with a bitter taste, was reported. These results suggest a possible role of heredity in the regulation of nutrient intake even though lifestyle and environmental factors contribute to the similarity observed within twin pairs.

We have also investigated the potential role of heredity on macronutrient selection and energy intake in a group of 375 families of the Quebec City area [11]. Data were available on 9 different kinds of relatives by descent or by adoption. As expected, significant familial resemblance accounting for about 30–40% of the variance was observed for energy and macronutrient intakes. The familial resemblance noted for energy intake was largely explained by environmental conditions and lifestyle characteristics shared by family members. This was also true for familial resemblance in macronutrient intake. However, we found evidence for a relatively minor genetic effect (about 20%) in the determination of individual differences in the proportion of energy derived from lipids and carbohydrates.

The observation of a potential role of heredity on macronutrient preference is not without raising the possibility that food choice may be involved in determining the inherited susceptibility of some people to obesity. This observation would certainly be compatible with the data indicating an increased preference for lipids in obese and postobese subjects in comparison to lean controls [12].

Pattern of Substrates Oxidized

In the context of the model presented here, the possibility of inherited differences in the pattern of substrate oxidation under standardized conditions is also a relevant issue. This can be indirectly assessed using the RQ as an indicator of the relative proportion of fat or carbohydrates oxidized provided testing conditions are carefully standardized and a few assumptions are made. Variation in substrate oxidation may be important in terms of weight or fat gain. Thus, 24-hour RQ measured in a metabolic chamber was recently shown to account for about 7% of the variance of weight gain over a period of about 2 years in male and female Pima indians [13]. In this case, those who were oxidizing relatively more carbohydrates than lipids were more at risk even though the overall effect was rather small.

Our recent report that RQ during submaximal exercise is less variable in identical twins than among fraternal twins suggests that there may be inherited differences in the predisposition to oxidize relatively more lipids or carbohydrates [14]. This finding has been reinforced by unpublished observations from our long-term overfeeding study. Indeed, we found a significant within-pair resemblance (within genotype) for the changes in RQ, at rest and for the next 4 h following a mixed meal challenge, as a result of chronic exposure to overfeeding over a period of 100 days. These results indicate that there are individuals prone to oxidize more fat than carbohydrates even when energy intake, macronutrient composition of the diet and the level of physical activity were standardized for more than 3 months. The twin resemblance observed in this study, particularly in terms of the response to overfeeding, suggests that genes have something to do with this phenomenon.

Over a period of several years, 26 pairs of identical twins were trained in our laboratory with standardized endurance and high-intensity cycle exercise programs for periods of 15–20 weeks. After 10 weeks of training, the twins were exercising 5 times per week, 45 min per session at the same relative intensity in each program. These training programs caused significant increases in maximal O_2 uptake and other indicators of aerobic performance. They were also associated with a decrease in the cardiovascular and metabolic response at a given submaximal power output. For instance, when exercising in relative steady state at 50 watts, there were decreases in heart rate, oxygen uptake, pulmonary ventilation, ventilatory equivalent of oxygen and in RQ with an increase in the oxygen pulse. For the particular case of RQ, in spite of the fact that twins were subjected to similar training regimens, individuals with the same genotypes were more similar in the changes with training for the pattern of relative substrate oxidized at a low power output level [15].

Skeletal Muscle Oxidative Potential

The ability of the skeletal muscle tissue to oxidize lipid substrates is correlated with the pattern of substrates oxidized in a variety of conditions. We have investigated the histochemical and biochemical characteristics of that tissue, using data obtained through biopsy of the vastus lateralis muscle in 32 pairs of brothers, 26 pairs of DZ and 35 pairs of MZ twins [16]. The heritability of the fiber type distribution and fiber areas was very low and nonsignificant.

The importance of the interindividual variability in the enzyme activity profile of human skeletal muscle confirms that one may find high and low activity levels of enzyme markers involved in the catabolism of different substrates in the skeletal muscle of healthy sedentary and moderately active individuals of both genders [17]. Numerous factors are undoubtedly involved in accounting for such large interindividual variations. Exercise-training is known to influence the enzyme activity level of human skeletal muscle [18], but only few studies have attempted to determine the heritability for different markers of the human skeletal muscle energy metabolism. In order to estimate the contribution of genetic factors, maximal enzyme activity of creatine kinase, hexokinase, phosphofructokinase (PFK), lactate dehydrogenase, malate dehydrogenase, 3-hydroxyacyl CoA dehydrogenase, and oxoglutarate dehydrogenase (OGDH) were determined in brother, DZ twin, and MZ twin sibships [16]. Although MZ twins exhibited significant within-pair resemblance for all skeletal muscle enzyme activity levels ($0.30 \leq r \leq 0.68$), the often nonsignificant intraclass coefficients found in brothers and DZ twins suggested that variations in enzyme activities were highly related to common environmental conditions and nongenetic factors. However, genetic factors appeared to be responsible for about 25–50% of the total phenotypic variation in the activities of the regulatory enzymes of the glycolytic (PFK) and citric acid cycle (OGDH) pathways and in the variation of the oxidative to glycolytic activity ratio (PFK/OGDH ratio) when the data were adjusted for age and gender differences [16]. In another study [19], ultrastructural features of skeletal muscle samples were determined in 11 MZ and 6 DZ twin pairs. No gene-associated variation in the mitochondrial volume density, the ratio of mitochondrial volume to myofibril volume, and the internal and external surface densities of mitochondria were observed. These results indicate that variation in the enzyme activity profile and oxidative potential of human skeletal muscle, even among sedentary subjects, appears to be less dependent on genetic factors than on other types of determinants.

Several skeletal muscle characteristics exhibit within identical twin pair similarity in response to training and this was observed in different exercise training experiments. On the basis of these observations, interindividual variations in training responses have been partly ascribed to hereditary factors since individuals with the same genotype (i.e. monozygotic twins) showed about the same magnitude of changes, while individuals with different genotypes did not exhibit the same response pattern to exercise-training. The results available until now suggest that genetic influences on the phenotypic expression of most of the skeletal muscle proteins involved in energy metabolism can be accounted for by alterations in the regulatory processes of gene expression rather than exon polymorphisms [15].

Conclusion

In conclusion, we believe that most of the human variation in body energy content is not associated with genetic individuality. The same conclusion is applicable to several correlates and affectors of excessive body energy content for stature or obesity. From these data, prevention of obesity would seem to be a reasonable proposition. Even though much research is needed on this topic, currently available evidence, part of which was reviewed here, suggests that preventive strategies should include attempts at influencing energy intake, fat content of the diet, and level of habitual physical activity because of its influences on energy balance, pattern of substrate oxidation and perhaps nutrient partitioning.

References

1 Van Itallie TB, Yang MV, Heymsfield SB, et al: Height-normalized indices of the body's fat-free mass and fat mass: Potentially useful indicators of nutritional status. Am J Clin Nutr 1990;52:853–859.
2 Bouchard C: Current understanding of the etiology of obesity: Genetic and nongenetic factors. Am J Clin Nutr 1991;53:1561S–1565S.
3 Bray GA: In Cioffi LA, James WPT, Van Itallie TB (eds): The Inheritance of Corpulence. The Body Weight Regulatory System: Normal and Disturbed Mechanisms. New York, Raven Press, 1991, pp 185–195.
4 Pérusse L, Leblanc C, Bouchard C: Intergeneration transmission of physical fitness in the Canadian population. Can J Sport Sci 1988;13:8–14.
5 Bouchard C, Pérusse L, Leblanc C, et al: Inheritance of the amount and distribution of human body fat. Int J Obes 1988;12:205–215.
6 Bouchard C, Tremblay A, Després JP, et al: The genetics of body energy content and energy balance: An overview; in Bray GA, Ryan DH (eds): The Science of Food Regulation. Baton Rouge, Louisiana State University Press, 1992, in press.
7 Bouchard C, Tremblay A, Després JP, et al: The response to long-term overfeeding in identical twins. N Engl J Med 1990;302:1477–1482.
8 Wade J, Milner J, Krondl M: Evidence for a physiological regulation of food selection and nutrient intake in twins. Am J Clin Nutr 1981;34:143–147.
9 Fabsitz RR, Garrison RJ, Feinleib M, et al: A twin analysis of dietary intake: evidence for a need to control for possible environmental differences in MZ and DZ twins. Behav Genet 1978;8:15–25.
10 Krondl M, Coleman P, Wade J, et al: A twin study examining the genetic influence on food selection. Hum Nutr 1983;37A:189–198.
11 Pérusse L, Tremblay A, Leblanc C, et al: Familial resemblance in energy intake: Contribution of genetic and environmental factors. Am J Clin Nutr 1988;47:629–635.
12 Drewnowski A, Greenwood MRC: Cream and sugar: Human preferences for high-fat foods. Physiol Behav 1983;30:629–633.
13 Zurlo F, Lilioja S, Esposito-Del Puente A, et al: Low ratio of fat to carbohydrate oxidation as predictor of weight gain. Am J Physiol 1990;259:E650–E657.
14 Bouchard C, Tremblay A, Nadeau A, et al: Genetic effect in resting and exercise metabolic rates. Metabolism 1989;38:364–370.

15 Bouchard C, Dionne FT, Simoneau JA, et al: Genetics of aerobic and anaerobic performances; in Holloszy JO (ed): Exercise and Sport Sciences Reviews. Baltimore, Williams & Wilkins, 1992, vol 20, in press.
16 Bouchard C, Simoneau JA, Lortie G, et al: Genetic effects in human skeletal muscle fiber type distribution and enzyme activities. Can J Physiol Pharmacol 1986;64: 1245–1251.
17 Simoneau JA, Bouchard C: Human variation in skeletal muscle fiber type proportion and enzyme activities. Am J Physiol 1989;49:799–805.
18 Saltin B, Gollnick P: Skeletal muscle adaptability: significance for metabolism and performance; in Peachey LD, Adrian RH, Geiger SR (eds): Handbook of Physiology, Skeletal Muscle. Bethesda, American Physiological Society, 1983, sect 10, chap 19, pp 555–631.
19 Howald H: Ultrastructure and biochemical function of skeletal muscles in twins. Ann Hum Biol 1976;3:455–462.

Claude Bouchard, PhD, Physical Activity Sciences Laboratory, PEPS,
Laval University, Ste-Foy G1K 7P4 PQ (Canada)

Simopoulos AP (ed): Nutrition and Fitness in Health and Disease.
World Rev Nutr Diet. Basel, Karger, 1993, vol 72, pp 78–91

Obesity and Its Treatment by Diet and Exercise

Jana Pařízková

Biomedical Center, Faculty of Physical Education, 2nd Medical School,
Charles University, Prague, Czechoslovakia

Introduction

In both developed and developing countries, the increased food availability and sedentary life-styles have been generating conditions for the development of excess weight and enhanced deposition of fat. This trend, along with high-risk lifestyles (smoking and high alcohol intake), is modifying the causes of mortality resulting in increased premature disability and death. This is of particular concern to the countries of Eastern Europe.

Since the 1st International Conference on Nutrition and Fitness in 1988 much has changed in Czechoslovakia. Nevertheless, the nutritional problems along with obesity have persisted. As compared to Western countries, the health situation is still worse, especially in regard to morbidity and mortality from cardiovascular diseases [1]. Unbalanced diet, not corresponding to real needs of the human organism, higher prices of food in general (especially those for fruit, vegetables, high quality proteins, etc.), sedentary life style, special stress situations, etc., have resulted, inter alia, in the enhanced deposition of fat and are considered as factors contributing to this unfavorable health status of our population.

The analysis of the development of obesity, and the definition of suitable markers enabling an early diagnosis in the subjects at risk have been difficult until recently due to the lack of the generally consented criteria at different age groups and in different parts of the world. Obesity is characterized by an increased body mass index (BMI) above 26.1 kg/m^2, excessive increased proportion of depot fat, and special subcutaneous fat patterning. There is an urgent need for diagnosis of early stages of obesity, especially during childhood and adolescence, when the efficient intervention by diet and exercise could be the most effective. This applies both to the actual, but also to the delayed health consequences of excess fatness later in life [2, 5, 10].

Since the 1960s, the serum cholesterol levels have increased significantly in both children and adults in Czechoslovakia [3]. The prevalence of obesity (i.e. the number of subjects with BMI higher than 30) also increased [4].

Body Compositon and Subcutaneous Fat Patterning in Various Population Groups

In the preschool age group, obesity was found rarely in our children (2–3%) [2]. About 10–12% of schoolchildren have been usually classified as overweight, depending on the criteria used. Studies in larger population samples of children, using also BMI, have been undertaken only recently. In the adults the prevalence of BMI higher than 30 was about 11–12% in subjects 55–64 years of age (results of the measurements of a stratified sample from 6 districts in Bohemia) [4]. The prevalence of obesity tended to increase during the period 1985–1988 in each age group, and most significantly in the oldest group of men. In the whole sample, the percentage of subjects with BMI higher than 30 increased significantly from 19.9% up to 25.4% as compared to the year 1985 (n = 2,546) until 1988 (n = 2,765) [4].

Figures 1 and 2 show the changes of BMI along with the percentage of depot fat and the centrality index (defined as the ratio of subscapular to triceps skinfold thickness; table 1) in the groups of subjects with the adequate body weight at different ages (n = 4,258). In females the centrality index did not change in the adult and more advanced age (up to 1.0) as it did in males (2.3–2.4).

As shown by more detailed longitudinal growth study, in 41 boys followed from 10.770 until 17.774 years (body composition evaluated by densitometry), the percentage of depot fat decreased significantly, with some fluctuation of values during puberty [1, 2]. In addition to that, BMI

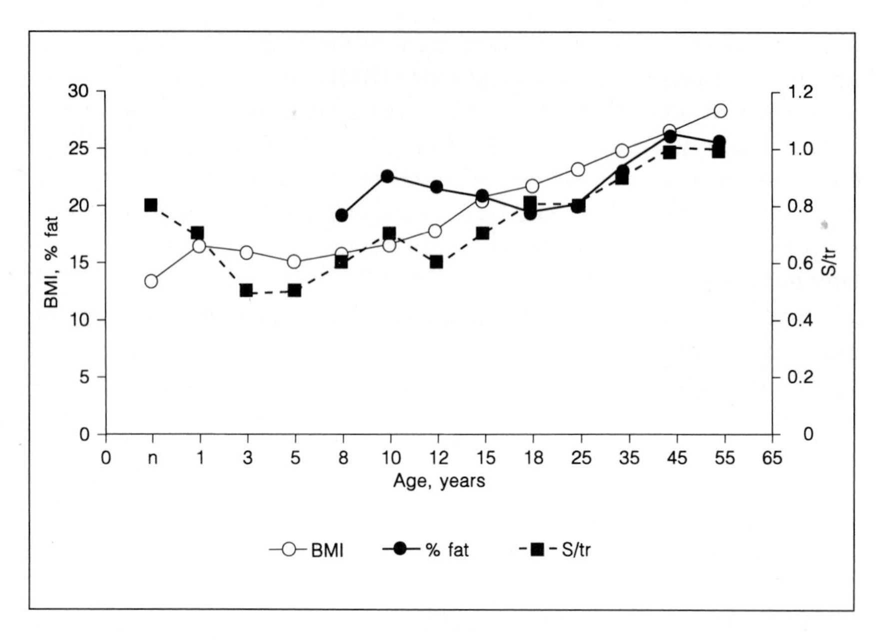

Fig. 1. Changes of body mass index (BMI), the percentage of body fat, and centrality index (ratio or subscapular/triceps skinfold thicknesses) in females during ontogeny.

Table 1. Developmental changes of centrality index (subscapular/triceps skinfold ratio) in boys followed longitudinally

Subject No.	Age years	Centrality index					Fat, %	
		25%	median	75%	$\bar{x}$	SD	$\bar{x}$	SD
1	10.770	0.56	0.62	0.79	0.70	0.21	16.0	5.1
2	11.744	0.56	0.64	0.73	0.69	0.24	15.0	7.0
3	12.681	0.62	0.71	0.84	0.81	0.32	14.4	5.9
4	13.741	0.83	1.00	1.19	1.01	0.33	11.1	5.3
5	14.641	0.73	0.85	1.00	0.89	0.26	13.1	4.7
6	15.741	0.82	1.00	1.38	1.09	0.38	12.9	5.2
7	16.799	0.88	1.00	1.33	1.11	0.32	11.1	4.0
8	17.774	0.93	1.11	1.39	1.17	0.32	9.0	4.8

Significance of differences was evaluated by Kruskall-Wallis one-way analysis of variance, and Kruskal-Wallis H (equivalent to chi square).

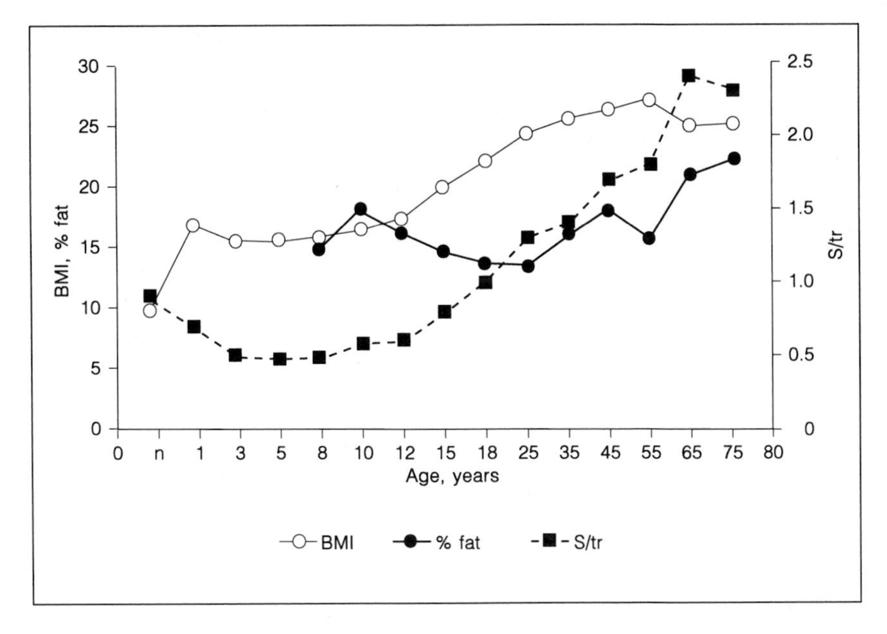

Fig. 2. Changes of body mass index (BMI), the percentage of body fat, and centrality index (ratio of subscapular/triceps skinfolds) in males during ontogeny.

increased significantly from 17.32 ± 1.63 up to 21.66 ± 2.13, and also the subcutaneous fat patterning changed significantly. There were only very small differences in the developmental trend of this index when comparing trained and control boys. In the obese adolescent boys this index was significantly higher (i.e. 2.45 ± 0.45).

The centrality index correlated significantly with the percentage of body fat only at the age of 12.681 years (r = 0.34, p at least 0.01) and with the absolute amount of fat (kg) at the same age (r = 0,38, p at least 0.01).

Indices, including more skinfolds on the trunk and the extremities, correlated more closely and significantly with depot fat. For example, the index relating the sum of skinfolds on the cheek, under chin, triceps, biceps, thigh and calf to the sum of skinfolds on the chest, abdomen, subscapular and suprailiac correlated significantly both with the relative [5] and absolute amount of depot fat (kg) (table 2). Thus, the analysis of the developmental changes during growth showed that in the individuals with lower amount of total body fat, the amount of subcutaneous fat on the extremities is relatively larger than that on the trunk. As apparent, fat patterning undergoes significant changes during adolescence in males along with the level of functional capacity [2].

Adult obese individuals (BMI around 40, the percentage of body fat before reduction treatment 35–40%; n = 84) had significantly higher value of this index, which was manifested more in males (2.31 ± 0.24) than in females (1.31 ± 0.06) [2].

Body Composition and Muscle Fiber Pattern

Lean body mass and depot fat is significantly related to a number of functional and morphological parameters which are associated with physical activity [1, 2]. For example, our last study showed a mild, but significant relationship of body components to muscle fiber pattern in a group of adult men, subdivided in control and athlete subgroups (table 3, 4) [6, 7]. This was manifested especially in the athletes, in which both body fat and

Table 2. Mean values of kg body fat index relating trunk/extremity skinfolds in adolescent boys followed longitudinally, and the correlation coefficients (r)

Subject No.	Fat, kg		Index		r
	$\bar{x}$	SD	$\bar{x}$	SD	
1	5.8	2.2	0.313	0.110	0.33*
2	6.0	3.1	0.217	0.068	0.70*
3	6.4	3.0	0.317	0.067	0.68*
4	5.6	3.3	0.330	0.051	0.80*
5	7.5	3.2	0.306	0.049	0.52*
6	8.5	3.0	0.333	0.047	0.56*
7	7.5	3.0	0.338	0.057	0.29
8	6.3	3.7	0.337	0.067	0.48*

Index = Sum of skinfolds on the chest, abdomen, subscapular, suprailiac/sum of skinfolds on the cheek, under chin, over triceps, biceps, thigh and calf.
Significance of differences was evaluated by Kruskall-Wallis one-way analysis of variance and Kruskall-Wallis H (equivalent to chi square).
* p at least 0.05.

muscle fiber pattern changed due to the adaptation to the dynamic exercise, resulting in lower BMI and decreased percentage of depot fat as well as low centrality index (0.8–1.2).

The percentage and the diameter of fast glycolytic fibers (FG), and the ratio of fast glycolytic to the sum of fast oxidative glycolytic (FOG) and

Table 3. Morphological and functional characteristics of men, experimental (athletes) and control [6, 7]

		Experimental (n = 106)	Control (n = 45)	Merged (n = 151)
Age , years	$\bar{x}$	21.38	26.8	23.00
	SD	4.14	8.0	6.7
Weight, kg	$\bar{x}$	74.8	71.64	73.8
	SD	11.87	7.15	10.77
Height, cm	$\bar{x}$	180.15	177.30	179.3
	SD	7.38	5.6	7.0
BMI	$\bar{x}$	22.9	22.7	22.9
	SD	2.6	1.9	2.4
Fat, %	$\bar{x}$	8.5	11.1	9.2
	SD	3.0	3.9	3.5
LBM, kg	$\bar{x}$	68.2	63.5	66.8
	SD	9.5	4.9	8.7
VO_2max	$\bar{x}$	58.00	51.66	56.1
	SD	10.1	9.0	10.2
FG, %	$\bar{x}$	23.72	24.37	23.91
	SD	16.07	13.47	15.31
FOG, %	$\bar{x}$	21.81	28.65	23.83
	SD	11.50	12.91	12.83
SO, %	$\bar{x}$	54.45	46.97	52.24
	SD	14.09	14.19	14.49
R1	$\bar{x}$	0.97	1.37	1.09
	SD	0.58	0.93	0.72
R2	$\bar{x}$	0.37	0.36	0.37
	SD	0.33	0.26	0.31

R1 = Ratio 1, FG + FOG/SO.
R2 = Ratio 2, FG/FOG + SO.

Table 4. The relationship between body composition and muscle fiber pattern (correlation coefficients r) [6, 7]

		FG %	FOG %	SO %	Ratio	FG diameter	SO diameter
BMI	Exp	0.281	0.214		0.283	0.249	0.219
	Sum	0.199	−0.179		0.205	0.216	0.196
LBM, %	Exp	0.237		0.209	−0.242		−0.198
	Sum			0.188			
LBM, kg	Exp	0.311	−0.211		0.316	0.247	
	Sum	0.223	−0.208		0.240	0.250	0.180
Fat, %	Exp	0.236		−0.209	0.242		0.198
	Sum			−0.188			
Fat, kg	Exp	0.313		−0.215	0.209	0.319	
	Sum	0.212		−0.198		0.210	

Ratio = FG/FOG + SO.
Exp (athletes, n = 106): p < 0.05–0.19, p < 0.01–0.25.
Sum (Exp + controls; n = 45): p < 0.05–0.16, p < 0.01–0.21.

slow oxidative (SO) fibers correlated most significantly with BMI and body composition in the group of athletes (runners) and/or in the merged group. The percentage of slow oxidative muscle fibers correlated significantly with the percentage of lean body mass, and negatively with the relative and absolute amount of body fat, indicating that the higher the proportion of slow oxidative muscle fibers, the lower the body fat; this manifested more markedly in the athletes adapted to dynamic exercise (table 4) [6, 7].

Similar relationships and changes of body composition along with muscle fiber pattern may appear also in other population groups, e.g. during exercise therapy in the obese.

Body Composition and Subcutaneous Fat Patterning in Vegetarians

Vegetarian diet has a marked impact on body composition and fat patterning similar to exercise. Measurements in adult vegetarians of both sexes in the fourth decade of life showed adequate values of BMI (males

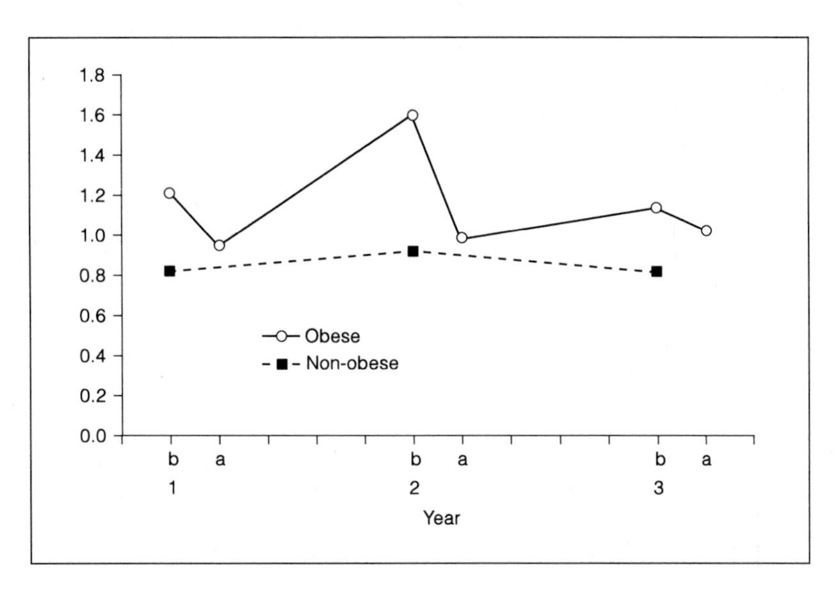

Fig. 3. Changes of the centrality index (ratio of subscapular/triceps skinfolds) in obese girls after repeated reduction treatment during a 3-year period. b = Before; a = after.

24.17 ± 2.27; females 21.81 ± 2.18) and of depot fat (males 14.4 ± 3.7%, females 21.4 ± 6.6%). No vegetarian was obese in our groups. Centrality index was slightly lower in males (1.42 ± 0.31), and the same in females (0.84 ± 0.23) as compared to subjects eating the usual mixed diet (fig. 1, 2) [8]. Vegetarian diet thus results in an adequate body mass index and fatness, as well as centrality index; it may help, even when introduced only partly, to reduce excess fatness in a population with an increased prevalence of obesity as ours [4].

Changes of Body Composition and Fat Patterning After Reduction Treatment by Diet and Exercise in the Obese

Figures 3 and 4 show the significant changes of the centrality index in the adolescent obese boys and girls treated during three years repeatedly in special summer camps by a monitored diet (7,530 kJ/day) and exercise regimens [2, 10]. Simultaneously, body weight decreased always by about

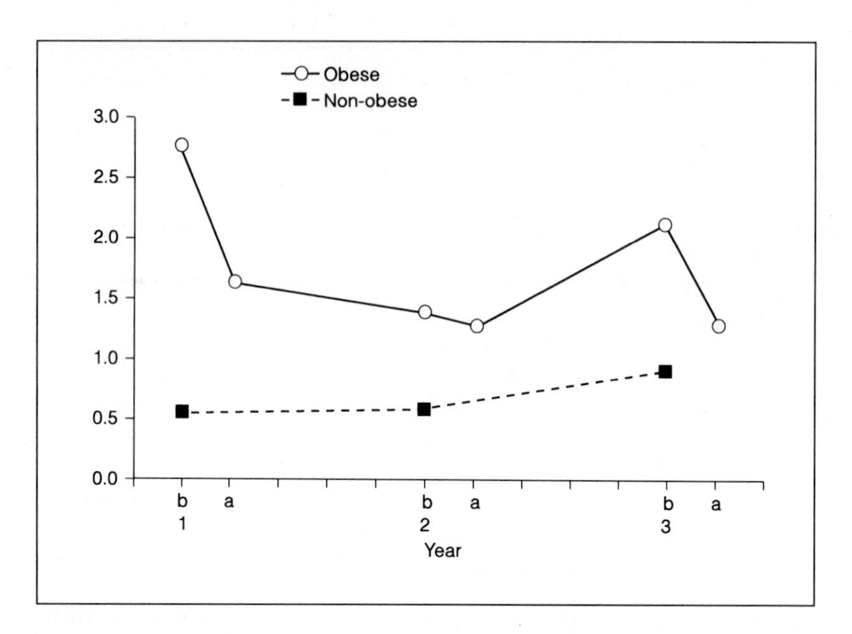

Fig. 4. Changes of the centrality index (ratio of subscapular/triceps skinfolds) in obese boys during a 3-year period.

10% of the initial value, and so did BMI. The level of functional capacity as tested by oxygen ceiling measurements, reaction to a standard work load, and physical fitness testing using various sport disciplines (running, broad jump, skill tests [2]) improved significantly [2, 9, 10] along with the above-mentioned changes of subcutaneous fat distribution. The changes in the fat patterning seem to be related also to the improvement of the functional capacity in weight reducing obese youth.

In the obese adult, treated with a low-energy diet (table 5) [5, 11] and an adjusted exercise program (30-min sessions of aerobic gymnastics, 15-min bouts of cycling on a cycle ergometer three times per day, with individual modifications, and 2 h walking at an intensity to increase the heart rate up to 130 beats/min [5, 10, 11]) for 4 weeks, a significant reduction of body weight was observed (by 8.5–15% of the initial value) along with a decrease in BMI, blood lipids, blood pressure, etc. [10, 11]. Nevertheless, even after this treatment a considerable degree of overweight still persisted. Centrality index did not change after this treatment (males before treatment 2.31 ± 0.24, after 2.34 ± 0.21; females before 1.31 ± 0.06, after

Table 5. Composition of low-energy diet (Dairy Research Institute. Prague) [5, 11]

Proteins	36.0 g
Carbohydrate	50.0 g
Fat	3.0 g
Energy content	1,555.0 kJ
Vitamins	Recommended dietary allowances, mmol
Na	39.1
K	48.6
Cl	56.4
Ca	31.0
P	32.3
Mg	14.4

1.32 ± 0.06). Also waist/hip ratio did not change after this short and efficient treatment (males before 1.02 ± 0.01, after 1.01 ± 0.01; females 0.87 ± 0.003, after 0.85 ± 0.01) similarly as waist/thigh ratio [11]. Also the aerobic power did not change after this treatment [12].

Fat Patterning in Females with Complicated Obesity

The analysis of the subcutaneous fat distribution of obese women with simple and complicated obesity showed significant differences. Figure 5 shows the comparison of total body fat, skinfold thickness and fat patterning in the adult women with BMI 24.78 (mean age 36.5 years) and normal percentage of body fat (N) as compared to standards of our population (fig. 1), than in women with simple, diffuse obesity (O) (BMI = 34.92, mean age 36.7 years), and finally women with disproportional (D), 'spider-like' [13] obesity (BMI = 30.77, mean age 36.0 years) which was accompanied by various metabolic diseases such as diabetes, hypercholesterolemia, etc. [13]. There were no significant differences in BMI and the amount of total body fat between the group of women with diffuse and disproportional, complicated obesity, which both differed in this respect significantly from group N. But the difference in fat patterning (as expressed by an

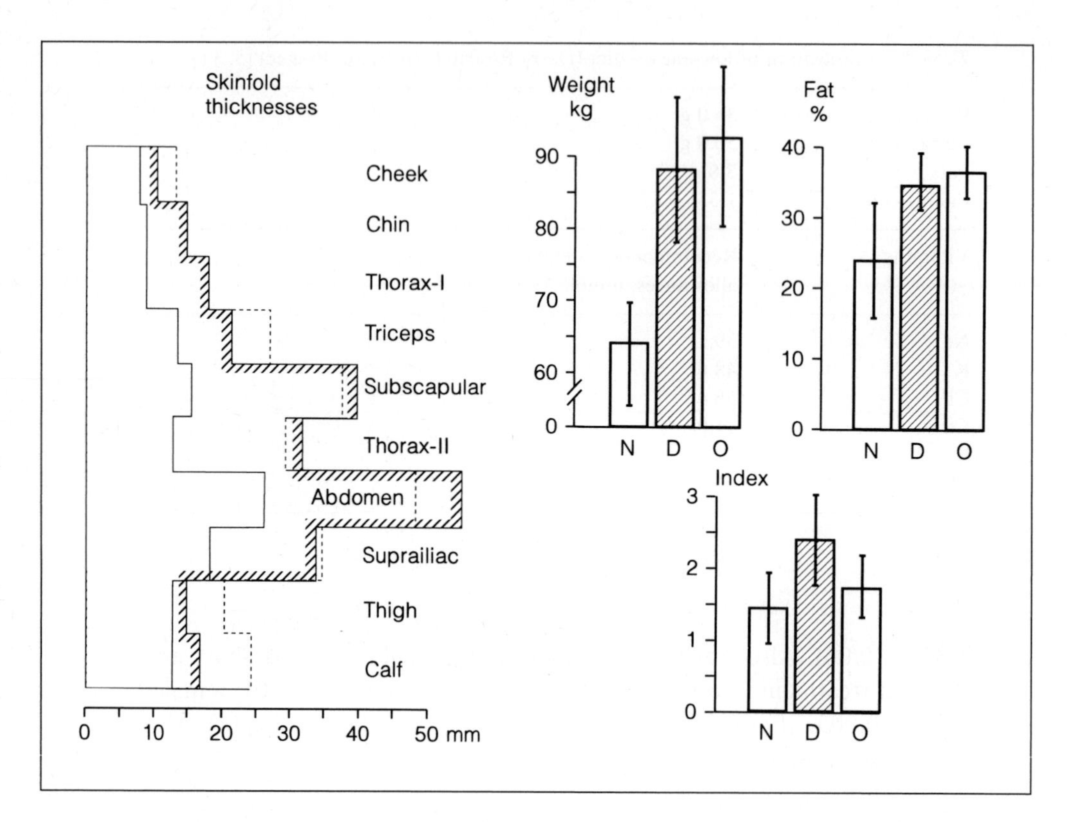

Fig. 5. The comparison of women with simple, diffuse obesity (O), women with disproportional obesity (D), and women with normal weight (n) as regards ten skinfold thicknesses, the percentage of depot fat measured by densitometry, and the index relating the sum of skinfolds on the trunk (subscapular, thorax, abdomen) and the sum of skinfolds on the extremities (triceps, biceps, thigh and calf). Based on the data of Skamenová and Pařízková [13].

index relating skinfold thicknesses on the trunk and the extremities) was highly significant [13]. The centrality index was 1.74 ± 0.48 in O, and 2.39 ± 0.51 in D; in control women with normal weight it was 1.41 ± 0.56.

It was most difficult to reduce excess weight and fat in the patients with disproportionate obesity (D) by dietary restriction and increased physical activity. Simultaneous treatment of accompanying illnesses was of course indispensable. In addition, the results of reducing therapy in subgroup D were not permanent, and reestablishment of the initial degree of obesity was more frequent than in simple obesity.

Conclusions

The last group of obese women characterized by disproportionate subcutaneous fat patterning and additional health problems (D) belonged to the worst cases of obesity as regards the possibility of the reduction treatment by exercise and diet. In similar cases performed later on [2, 5, 11, 12] it has been always very difficult to help by exercise and diet only, in spite of the fact that they have always been useful factors for the rectification of excess fatness. A special individual approach to reduction treatment was indispensable, and the results of the treatment were mostly nonlasting.

In the adult obese, in which simple diffuse obesity is diagnosed, exercise and diet therapy can lead to long-lasting improvements. At this age it is possible to use more radical diet, as, e.g., VLCD described above (table 5) [5, 11]. But at the beginning there have always been difficulties with exercise, as in the obese with BMI higher than 35–40. The introduction of necessarily intensive exercise of dynamic character may be very problematic because of the lowered functional capacity and cardiorespiratory efficiency, joint and vertebral column problems, etc. In the morbid cases of obesity, only mild selected exercise (e.g. spa treatment in the swimming pool, in the lying position, etc.) may be introduced gradually, with permanent medical supervision. Only later after some reduction of body weight, BMI and fat, the intensity of exercise, preferably of the dynamic character, may be possible. Such a regimen must be adhered to permanently, along with the adequately reduced dietary intake and overall adjusted way of life. Otherwise, the return to the initial degree of obesity has been always noticed [5, 10–12].

During adolescence, on the contrary, exercise is primarily the best way of obesity treatment. Adaptation to a more intensive physical activity regimen is more easily possible. In the cases of morbid obesity, again, the gradual introduction of mild exercise as mentioned above could be used at the beginning of the reduction treatment. In contrast with the adult obese, strictly reduced dietary intake is not recommended, as it is necessary to assure, even during the reduction of excess fat, an optimal growth in height, and also further adequate somatic and functional development. Growth retardation, decrease of lean body mass (undesirable during growth [2], but eventually tolerable in adult age [5, 10, 11]), and of the functional capacity were observed, when diet of only 4,182 kJ (1,000 kcal) per day was introduced [2]. In growing individuals the dietary intake has to be very carefully monitored individually, based on the recommendations of the World Health Organization [14].

The best treatment of the obesity problem is of course its prevention, started as early as possible. Spontaneous physical activity decreases significantly at the beginning of school as compared to preschool age, not only during school hours, but also during leisure time [10].

Under conditions of life in the developed countries, but also in the well-off social strata in the developing countries, it is indispensable to monitor the regimen of physical activity and nutrition at a very early age. This concerns especially those children at greater risk of an easy increase of body weight and fat (e.g. due to family history), and arrange for them also the opportunity for spontaneous physical exercise as well as suitable physical education (e.g. special exercises of children with their parents [2]). Overeating ought to be prevented as early as possible.

Diet and exercise limiting obesity are also the best factors decreasing the risk of cardiovascular diseases later in life: the prevention could be most effective when started as early as possible, as stated also in the Document of the World Health Organization on 'Prevention in childhood of cardiovascular diseases later in life' [15]. Thus, exercise and diet can help not only against excess fatness, but also as a preventive factor against coronary heart disease, the greatest killer in the developed countries. The selection of the individuals at risk can be facilitated by using simple markers [16, 17] such as family history and fat distribution. Up to now, this risk has been greater in Eastern Europe, to which greater attention ought to be paid, not only for health and humanitarian reasons, but also from the point of view of necessary economic development in the future.

References

1 Pařízková J: Nutrition and exercise as a way for controlling aging. Coll Anthrop 1990;14:203–316.

2 Pařízková J: Body Fat and Physical Fitness. The Hague, Martinus Nijhoff BV/Medical Division, 1977.

3 Pistulková H, Poledne R, Kautská J, Škodová Z, Petržiková Z, Paclt M, Valenta Z, Grafnetter D, Píša Z: Cholesterolemia in school age children and hypercholesterolemia in family aggregation. Cor Vasa 1991;33:139–149.

4 Škodová Z, Píša Z, Berka L, Cícha Z, Eurová R, Pithartová J, Vorlíček J, Wiesner E, Vojtíšek P, Petržilková Z, Čeřovská J, Valenta Z: The development of body weight in population of Czech republic (in Czech). Čas Lék Čes. 1990;129:1033–1035.

5 Hainer V, Kunešová M, Štich V, Pařízková J, Žák A, Malec B: Long-term follow-up of obese patients treated initially by very low calorie diet (VLCD). Int J Obesity 1991;15(suppl):30.
6 Melichna J, Zauner G, Pařízková J, Havlíčková L: Relationship of muscle fibre distribution to body composition in physically trained and normally active human males (abstract). Med Sci Sports Exerc 1992;2(Suppl):16.
7 Melichna J, Pařízková J, Zauner C, Havlíčková L: Relationship of muscle fiber distribution to body composition in physically trained and normally active human males. Am J Hum Biol, in press.
8 Pařízková J: Adaptation of functional capacity to exericse; in Baxter, Waterlaw JC (eds): Nutritional Adaptation in Man. London, Libbey, 1985, pp 127–139.
9 Pařízková J: Age-dependent changes in dietary intake related to work output, physical fitness, and body composition. Am J Clin Nutr 1989;49:962–967.
10 Pařízková J, Hainer V: Exercise in growing and adult obese individuals; in Torg JS, Welsh RP, Shephard RJ (eds): Current Therapy in Sports Medicine-2. Toronto, Decker 1990, pp 22–27.
11 Hainer V, Štich V, Kunešová M, Pařízková J, Žák A, Wernischová V, Štukavec V: Body fat distribution, metabolic and hormonal indices in obese patients treated initially by very low calorie diet; in: Diet and Obesity, Tokyo/Basel, Japan Science Society Press/Karger, 1991, pp 17–28.
12 Štich V, Hainer V, Kunešová M, Malec B, Peslarová J: Has VLCD the impact on the tolerance of the work load? (in Czech). Čas Lék Čes, in press.
13 Skamenová B, Pařízková J: Assessment of disproportional (spiderlike) and diffuse type of obesity by measurement of the total and subcutaneous body fat (in Czech). Čas Lék Čes 1963;102:142–146.
14 Energy and Protein Requirements: Report of a Joint FAO/WHO/UNU Expert Consultation. Tech Rep Ser 724. Geneva, World Health Organization, 1985.
15 Prevention in Childhood and Youth of Adult Cardiovascular Diseases: Time for Action. Report of a WHO Expert Committee. Tech Rep Ser 792. Geneva, World Health Organization, 1990.
16 Bouchard C, Johnston FE (eds): Fat Distribution during Growth and Later Health Outcomes. New York, Liss, 1988.
17 Olsen RE, Beutler E, Broquist HP: Physiologic basis for the control of body fat distribution in humans. Ann Rev Nutr 1989;9:417–443.

Jana Pařízková, MD, PhD, DSc, Biomedical Center,
Faculty of Physical Education, 2nd Medical School, Charles University,
J. Martiho 31, 16252 Prague 6 (Czechoslovakia)

Panel V
Osteoporosis

Simopoulos AP (ed): Nutrition and Fitness in Health and Disease.
World Rev Nutr Diet. Basel, Karger, 1993, vol 72, pp 92–101

Local and Systemic Factors in the Pathogenesis of Osteoporosis

Lawrence G. Raisz

University of Connecticut Health Center, Farmington, Conn., USA

Introduction

In order to fulfill its dual functions as a storehouse for mineral and as the structural framework of the body, the skeleton must be regulated by both systemic hormones and local factors. Osteoporosis is a common disorder, or family of disorders, in which skeletal mass and strength decrease resulting in an increased propensity for fractures. The pathogenesis of osteoporosis is currently unknown and almost certainly multifactorial [1]. Moreover, there are multiple osteoporotic syndromes with different clinical and morphologic features which probably have different pathogenetic mechanisms. These pathogenetic mechanisms can all be considered as representing failure of normal coupled bone turnover. In the adult skeleton, bone formation is coupled to bone resorption. Remodeling occurs at both trabecular and cortical sites and continues throughout life. Bone loss in osteoporosis can result from several different combinations of changes in bone resorption and formation. Accelerated bone resorption will lead to an initial bone loss simply because there are more resorption cavities present, but if the capacity for bone formation is unimpaired, then these cavities will be filled and a new steady state achieved. However, accelerated resorption will also cause loss of template, in particular, trabecular bone plates may be completely removed so that no new bone formation can occur. Even if bone resorption is not accelerated, bone loss will occur if bone formation is impaired. It is likely that both increased resorption and decreased formation occur in most forms of osteoporosis.

There are four groups of agents which are likely to be involved in pathogenesis: (1) the calcium-regulating hormones; parathyroid hormone (PTH), 1,25-dihydroxyvitamin D ($1,25(OH)_2D$) and calcitonin (CT); (2) the systemic growth-regulating hormones: growth hormone, glucocorticoids, thyroid hormone and sex hormones; (3) the local stimulators of bone resorption: prostaglandins, particularly PGE_2, and cytokines, particularly interleukin-1 (IL-1); (4) the local regulators of bone formation: insulin-like growth factors I and II (IGF-I and IGF-II), transforming growth factor β (TGFβ) and the bone morphogenetic proteins (BMP). These are by no means the only potential pathogenetic factors in osteoporosis. Other cytokines and growth factors have been implicated.

However, this review will focus on the mode of action on the skeleton and the possible roles in osteoporosis of the agents listed above.

Parathyroid Hormone

The most important physiologic function of PTH is to maintain serum ionized calcium concentration. This is accomplished by stimulation of bone resorption, distal tubular reabsorption of calcium in the kidney and increased synthesis of $1,25(OH)_2D_3$, which in turn results in increased intestinal calcium absorption. The phosphaturic action of PTH supports this function by facilitating bone resorption, enhancing $1,25(OH)_2D_3$ synthesis and preventing redeposition of calcium with phosphate in bone and soft tissue. However, PTH has many other actions on the skeleton. In mild primary hyperparathyroidism and in patients given intermittent injections of PTH, there is an increase in trabecular bone mass, although cortical bone mass is either unaffected or decreased [2]. The fact that intermittent PTH can increase trabecular bone mass has actually been used as therapy in osteoporosis.

This effect may not be due to a direct action of PTH, since PTH inhibits osteoblastic collagen synthesis in vitro. There is evidence that PTH can increase the production of IGF-I by bone (see below), as well as active TGFβ [3]. Other growth factors may also be involved.

Both excess and deficiency of PTH have been implicated as pathogenetic mechanisms in osteoporosis. In women with vertebral crush fractures, the PTH response to a hypocalcemic stimulus of phosphate loading is blunted [4]. This could either represent an intrinsic defect in the function of the parathyroid glands or could be due to the fact that other factors which stimulate bone resorption have replaced the parathyroids, and they are less responsive. In older individuals with age related calcium deficiency, due both to impairment of intestinal absorption and decreased renal synthesis of 1,25$(OH)_2$D, secondary hyperparathyroidism probably occurs. In any event, there is definitely an age related increase in PTH. Whether or not these high PTH levels are correlated with decreased bone mass has not been established.

1,25-Dihydroxyvitamin D

The major function of 1,25$(OH)_2$D in adults is to maintain the supply of calcium and phosphate by stimulating intestinal absorption [5]. With dietary calcium or phosphate deficiency, 1,25$(OH)_2$D levels increase substantially. Under these conditions, increased intestinal absorption is not the primary target, but stimulation of bone resorption and inhibition of formation occurs. Thus 1,25$(OH)_2$D helps to maintain the supply of minerals to soft tissues by removing them from bone. Vitamin D is important in cellular differentiation. 1,25$(OH)_2$D is required for the formation of osteoclasts and the differentiated function of osteoblasts. Thus, it is possible that when vitamin D levels are low, bone remodeling is impaired.

Vitamin D deficiency or impaired synthesis of 1,25$(OH)_2$D have been implicated in the pathogenesis of age related bone loss. Although classically vitamin D deficiency is associated with osteomalacia, low levels of the precursor 25-hydroxyvitamin D as well as 1,25$(OH)_2$D have been described in patients with hip fractures with osteoporosis rather than the impaired mineralization characteristic of osteomalacia. 1,25$(OH)_2$D as well as other vitamin D metabolites have been used widely in the treatment of osteoporosis. One recent study suggests that small doses of calcitriol will decrease the incidence of vertebral fractures in postmenopausal women [6]. 1,25$(OH)_2$D being the hormonal form is potentially more toxic, and precursor forms such as 1α-hydroxyvitamin D are widely used. Other forms of vitamin D which might have selective anabolic effects on bone are currently under study.

Calcitonin

When CT was discovered to be a potent inhibitor of bone resorption 30 years ago, it was considered likely that deficiency of this hormone would be an important pathogenetic mechanism in osteoporosis and that it would be an effective therapeutic agent. The former does not appear to be the case, although the latter has been amply demonstrated. Most studies measuring CT levels in patients with vertebral crush fracture syndrome or in older individuals with hip fracture do not show any deficiency. Moreover, the response of CT to a hypercalcemic stimulus is not blunted in osteoporotic patients. Nevertheless, calcitonin is clearly a potent inhibitor of bone resorption when given in pharmacologic doses. It is widely used in the treatment of osteoporosis, particularly in those with high bone turnover. Recent studies have suggested that CT may also stimulate bone formation. Further studies are needed, since many analogs of calcitonin are available for testing and any selective effect on bone formation would be most useful clinically.

Growth Hormone

While GH is the major regulator of somatic growth, it probably acts indirectly by stimulating the production of circulating and local IGFs [7]. Since skeletal tissue can produce abundant amounts of IGF, probably mainly in the form of IGF-II, and growth hormone can stimulate this production, circulating IGF may be of less importance for bone. GH deficiency is associated with impaired growth in children, but it is not clear that GH deficiency results in decreased bone mass in adults. There is an age-related decrease in the pulsatile secretion of GH and circulating levels of IGF-I. Interpretation of effects on IGF, both in the circulation and in the target tissues, is complicated by the fact that the binding proteins for IGF are also regulated. There are at least six IGF binding proteins. Most probably inhibit IGF action, but some may enhance the response.

While circulating IGF-I is probably not decreased in patients with osteoporosis, impairment of local production or increased production of inhibitory binding proteins could be a pathogenetic mechanism. IGF probably does play a role in mediating the impaired bone formation in glucocorticoid-induced osteoporosis and may also mediate anabolic responses to sex hormones.

Glucocorticoids

The effects of glucocorticoids on skeletal tissue are complex [8]. Glucocorticoids have both direct and indirect effects on the skeleton. Among the most important indirect effects are inhibition of calcium absorption in the intestine and of GH secretion by the pituitary. Although the direct effect of glucocorticoid excess is to decrease DNA and protein synthesis in bone, glucocorticoids may enhance bone cell differentiation and increase the response to other local and systemic hormones, including PTH and IGFs. Glucocorticoids may act by decreasing local IGF-I production. They also decrease the production of PGE_2 and IL-1. On the other hand, both PGE_2 and IL-1 can have anabolic effects on bone in the presence of glucocorticoids at concentrations which are catabolic in their absence.

Although there is no question that excess glucocorticoids can produce osteoporosis, it is not clear whether increased bone resorption or decreased bone formation is the more important pathogenetic mechanism. Much of the data favor decreased bone formation as the more important, but therapeutic approaches have largely been aimed at decreasing bone resorption. An early approach was to attempt to overcome the impaired calcium absorption by calcium and vitamin D loading. This had some effect on bone mass but does not reverse osteoporosis in glucocorticoid-treated patients. Increased bone mass can occur after treatment with calcitonin and bisphosphonates which inhibit bone resorption, but increases are also observed with fluoride therapy which stimulates bone formation. There are some recent studies which suggest that different glucocorticoids with similar anti-inflammatory potency may differ in their tendency to produce osteoporosis, but this has not been clearly established.

Thyroid Hormones

Thyroid hormones are probably essential for cartilage and bone growth as well as for bone turnover. Both T_4 and T_3 have been shown to stimulate bone resorption both by prostaglandin-dependent and prostaglandin-independent mechanisms in different organ culture systems. Bone formation is increased secondary to this increase in resorption, but excessive thyroid hormones usually results in bone loss.

The importance of thyroid hormones in the pathogenesis of osteoporosis remains controversial. There are a number of studies suggesting that thyroid hormone replacement in hypothyroid patients can result in bone loss and that patients with hyperthyroidism who are treated with excessive doses of exogenous thyroid hormone have decreased bone mass [9]. However, not all studies confirm this. Many postmenopausal women are on replacement thyroid hormone therapy and excessive doses may be an aggravating factor in the development of osteoporosis.

Sex Hormones

Sex hormones, both estrogen and androgens, play a central role in skeletal development and bone loss. The increases in estrogen and testosterone as well as adrenal androgen at puberty are presumably responsible for a complex sequence of events involving first acceleration and then cessation of cartilage growth and an increase in bone turnover characterized by a greater rate of formation and a consequent increase in bone mass. Although early studies emphasize the possible role of calcium regulating and other systemic hormones in mediating the response to sex hormones, recent data have shown that the skeleton is affected more directly. With respect to calcium regulating hormones, estradiol (E_2) has been shown to increase vitamin D levels, probably by increasing the vitamin D-binding protein. Estrogen can decrease IGF-I production by the liver, and this in turn may lead to decreased feedback inhibition at the hypothalamus or pituitary, and hence increase pulsatile GH secretion.

The finding that estrogen and androgen receptors are present in bone cells under certain circumstances and recent studies showing direct effects of these hormones on isolated bone cell and organ cultures have pointed to a different mechanism of sex hormone action. E_2 and also testosterone (T) can inhibit prostaglandin production by bone [10, 11]. Macrophages from E_2-treated subjects also show decreased IL-1 production. In cell culture, increases in IGF and TGFβ have been observed. There may be additional effects of E_2 and T on bone cell metabolism independent of these mediators, but these have not yet been convincingly demonstrated.

The progressive bone loss that occurs after oophorectomy or orchidectomy or at the menopause appears to be due predominantly to an increase in bone resorption. The absolute rate of bone formation also increases, but the increase is relatively smaller than the increase in resorption. Thus, it seems reasonable to postulate that both E_2 and T have an anabolic effect on bone in addition to their anti-resorptive effect.

The importance of sex hormone deficiency in the pathogenesis of osteoporosis is well established. Hormone replacement therapy can block bone loss in postmenopausal or oophorectomized women and increase bone mass in hypogonadal men. However, there is a marked difference in rates of bone loss among hypogonadal individuals which does not always correlate with sex hormone levels. Whether there is a difference in end organ responsiveness to the sex hormones or whether there is a superimposed pathogenetic mechanism involving local factors remains to be determined.

Prostaglandins

Prostaglandins are complex, multifunctional regulators which are produced by bone cells and probably play an important role in local regulation [12]. Prostaglandin E_2 (PGE_2) and prostaglandin I_2 (PGI_2) are probably the most important endogenous regulators, although other prostanoids as well as lipoxygenase metabolites of arachidonic acid have effects on bone. PGE_2 and PGI_2 both stimulate bone resorption. This effect is relatively slow, involving the development of new osteoclasts, and may be preceded by a transient inhibition of the function of existing osteoclasts. The resorptive effect of prostaglandins probably is important in the bone loss of inflammation and in the early phases of immobilization. Exogenous prostaglandins have been shown to stimulate bone formation in animal models and in human infants. This effect may not be direct but may be mediated by an increased production of local growth factors. High concentrations of PGE_2 can inhibit osteoblastic collagen synthesis by a transcriptional effect. The relative importance of the stimulatory and inhibitory effects in vivo in response to changes in endogenous prostaglandin production is unknown.

Prostaglandin production in bone is highly regulated. Increased mechanical strain can increase PG production, and this may be one of the mechanisms by which mechanical forces influence bone remodeling. Most of the hormones which affect bone resorption and formation also affect prostaglandin synthesis. The relative importance of the PG response varies. For example, in different organ culture and in vivo studies, IL-1 has been shown to have both prostaglandin-dependent and prostaglandin-independent effects on bone resorption.

A role for prostaglandins in osteoporosis is suggested by the observation that bone PG production is increased in oophorectomized rats and decreased by estrogen administration both in vivo and in vitro.

Cytokines

IL-1 and tumor necrosis factor (TNF) have been shown to be powerful stimulators of bone resorption and inhibitors of bone formation [1]. Other cytokines such as IL-4, IL-6 and LIF have been found to act on bone, but the studies are conflicting. Colony-stimulating factors (CSF) also affect bone cell function. There is an M-CSF deficient mouse model of osteopetrosis in which osteoclast formation is restored by M-CSF treatment [13]. While most cytokines have been implicated as stimulators of bone resorption, interferon-γ is an inhibitor, which is particularly effective against cytokines but also blocks the effects of systemic stimulators.

The possibility that cytokine excess is responsible for bone loss in osteoporosis is supported by observations on the production of IL-1 and TNF by peripheral macrophages. Cytokine production is increased in macrophages from estrogen-deficient and osteoporotic subjects, and this is reversed by estrogen therapy. It is possible that this change in macrophages is due to activation by fragments of resorbing bone, rather than representing a primary pathogenetic mechanism. The fact that patients with multiple myeloma can show a severe form of vertebral crush fracture syndrome, which is reversed when their disease is controlled, supports a pathogenetic role for cytokines. Myeloma cells produce IL-1 and TNFβ, both of which are potent bone resorbers.

Growth Factors

Both IGF-1 and IGF-II are produced by bone and their production is regulated by systemic and local factors [14]. The IGFs cause an increase in the replication and differentiation of osteoblasts and are potent anabolic agents in the skeleton. Deficiency of IGF is clearly associated with decreased bone formation. Unlike many other growth factors, IGFs have little effect on bone resorption. Whether endogenous IGF production is important in the pathogenesis of osteoporosis remains to be proven.

TGFβ is a multifunctional regulator of many cell types and bone cells are no exception. TGFβ can inhibit bone resorption directly, although in some culture systems it produces prostaglandin-dependent stimulation. TGFβ is a potent mitogen for bone cells which also increases their differentiated function. Latent TGFβ in bone could be activated during the resorptive process and this could provide a mechanism for coupling, that is, it could stop osteoclastic resorption and initiate osteoblastic formation. However, the long lag between these two events during the reversal phase makes it difficult to assign them to a single factor. Bone contains a family of BMPs which bear some homology to TGFβ, but clearly have different effects. There are studies in which TGFβ has been less effective than BMPs in increasing bone formation in vivo. Here again, one can only speculate on pathogenetic roles for these substances. There is, of course, great interest in their possible therapeutic use for stimulating bone formation and healing bony defects, as well as treating osteoporosis.

Among the other bone growth factors, FGF is a potent mitogen which appears to inhibit collagen synthesis in cell and organ culture, while PDGF is mitogenic but does not inhibit collagen synthesis and may even increase osteoblast function.

Conclusions

This summary of the major local and systemic factors which influence bone metabolism points to the complexity of skeletal regulation and supports the concept that pathogenetic mechanisms in osteoporosis will be equally complex. In order to resolve these complex issues, it will be necessary to develop methods for assessing the local production of and response to these factors. New methods of molecular biology are currently being applied to these questions and should improve our understanding of the pathogenesis and consequently help us to develop more specific and effective therapies for this widespread disorder.

References

1 Raisz LG: Local and systemic factors in the pathogenesis of osteoporosis. N Engl J Med 1988;318:818–827.
2 Silverberg SJ, Shane E, De La Cruz L, et al: Skeletal disease in primary hyperparathyroidism. J Bone Miner Res 1989;283–291.
3 Canalis E, Centrella M, Burch W, et al: Insulin-like growth factor-1 mediates selective anabolic effects of parathyroid hormone in bone cultures. J Clin Invest 1989;83:60–65.
4 Silverberg JS, Shane E, Clemens TL, et al: The effect of oral phosphate administration on major indices of skeletal metabolism in normal subjects. J Bone Miner Res 1986;1:383–388.
5 Raisz LG: Recent advances in bone cell biology: Interactions of vitamin D with other local and systemic factors. Bone Mineral 1990;9:191–197.
6 Tilyard MW, Spears GFS, Thomson J, et al: Treatment of postmenopausal osteoporosis with calcitriol or calcium. N Engl J Med 1992;326:357–362.
7 Raisz LG, Kream BE: Regulation of bone formation. N Engl J Med 1983;309:29–35, 83–89.
8 Lukert BP, Raisz LG: Glucocorticoid-induced osteoporosis: Pathogenesis and management. Ann Intern Med 1990;112:352–364.

9 Kung AWC, Pun KK: Bone mineral density in premenopausal women receiving a long-term physiological dose of Levothyroxine. J Am Med Assoc 1991;265:2688–2691.
10 Pilbeam CC, Klein-Nulend J, Raisz LG: Inhibition by 17β-estradiol of PTH stimulated resorption and prostaglandin production in cultured neonatal mouse calvariae. Biochem Biophys Res Commun 1989;183:1319–1324.
11 Pilbeam CC, Raisz LG: Effects of androgens on parathyroid hormone and interleukin-1-stimulated prostaglandin production in cultured neonatal mouse calvariae. J Bone Miner Res 1990;5:1183–1188.
12 Raisz LG, Pilbeam CC, Klein-Nulend, J, et al: Prostaglandins and bone metabolism: Possible role in osteoporosis; in Christiansen C, Overgaard K (eds): Osteoporosis. Copenhagen, Osteopress, 1990, pp 253–258.
13 Felix R, Cecchini MG, Hofstetter W, et al: Impairment of macrophage colony-stimulating factor production and lack of resident bone marrow macrophages in the osteopetrotic op/op mouse. J Bone Miner Res 1990;5:781–789.
14 Canalis E, McCarthy T, Centrella M: Isolation of growth factors from adult bovine bone. Calcif Tissue Int 1988;43:346–351.

Lawrence G. Raisz, MD, University of Connecticut Health Center,
Farmington, CT 06030 (USA)

Simopoulos AP (ed): Nutrition and Fitness in Health and Disease.
World Rev Nutr Diet. Basel, Karger, 1993, vol 72, pp 102–113

Nutrition and Fitness in the Prophylaxis for Age-Related Bone Loss in Women

Lisbeth Nilas

Department of Clinical Chemistry, Glostrup Hospital, Glostrup, Denmark

In osteoporosis the amount of bone mineral per volume of bone tissue is reduced and the liability to fractures increased. The fractures occur primarily in the spine, forearm, hip and humerus and cause suffering and disability in the individual and large social expenses. Several factors determine the fracture risk, but the most important risk factor is a low bone mass. The structural and architectural changes in the bone framework of old osteoporotic bones implies that therapies restoring bone mass do not necessarily restore bone strength. Strategies towards prevention of fracture risk must therefore concentrate on increasing the maximal adult bone mass and preventing the age-related bone loss.

In females peak adult bone mass is reached during the third decade, but the individual variation in bone mass is large. Our knowledge about the factors regulating skeletal growth are limited. The peak bone mass depends on race and is under strong genetic influence, and is believed to be affected by nutrition and physical activity. Some studies have suggested that vertebral density declines during the premenopausal years, but more recent data have shown that bone mass in all skeletal regions is almost constant until the beginning of the menopausal transition. The majority of the life-time loss of bone occurs in relation to the menopause, where the cessation of ovarian function leads to increased bone resorption and bone loss. The declining bone mass follows an exponential curve with initial annual rates of loss of two to five percent. Immediately after the menopause, trabecular bone loss exceeds cortical, but the loss gradually declines and has ceased in most women by the age of 70 years. Some describe the pattern of bone loss in women as a slow age-related loss on which a faster, menopause-related loss is superimposed. Estrogen/progestogen replacement therapy is effective in preventing both the menopausal bone loss and subsequent fractures, and newer agents such as calcitonin and diphosphonates inhibit bone loss, but these treatments are not tolerated or wanted by all. There is increasing interest in the role of life-style factors on bone mass, but the widespread belief that keeping fit and supplementing the diet with calcium prevents osteoporotic fractures is not scientifically justified.

Bone Mass and Physical Activity

Experimental studies have shown that bones respond to stress and accommodate to the forces applied to them. Prolonged immobility or inactivity and the weightlessness experienced during astronaut flights causes negative calcium balance and a decline in bone mass predominantly in the lower extremities. An increased bone mass is found in the dominant arm of dedicated male and female tennis players. These observations indicate that bone mass can be modulated by physical activity, and weight-bearing exercises are suggested in the prevention of osteoporosis. We now have a large amount of data on bone mass in young athletic women, but the effects of exercise on bones are difficult to interpret because of the frequent occurrence of contemporary menstrual disturbances. The results from epidemiological data are somewhat conflicting and most longitudinal studies are not randomized and have a short duration.

Exercise-Induced Amenorrhea

Premature estrogen deficiency as seen after surgical oophorectomy is associated with premature bone loss and increased risk of osteoporosis. Women with secondary amenorrhea have a bone deficit of 15–30% in the vertebras and a smaller deficit in peripheral bones [1, 2]. The bone deficit occurs in both hyperprolactinemic and hypothalamic amenorrhea and in premature ovarian failure, and is not related to the cause of the condition, but to the duration and severity of the estrogen deficiency [1, 2]. Studies from recent years have shown that menstrual disorders as oligomenorrhea, luteal phase insufficiency and anovulation also have adverse effects on the skeleton [3]. Exercise-induced amenorrhea is now accepted as a clinical diagnosis. The endocrine profile is that of hypothalamic amenorrhea with low estrogen concentrations and elevated gonadotropins, but the pathogenesis is not fully understood. The condition is especially seen in endurance sports such as running and dancing. Development of athletic amenorrhea or other menstrual disturbances is associated with the training frequency and intensity, the age at menarche, a low body weight and a low fat to lean tissue ratio. Eating disturbances are also a common finding. Early intensive training may retard the menarche and increase the risk of secondary amenorrhea. In the amenorrheic athlete the menses will often reappear after a gain in weight and reduction of training intensity, changes that typically occur during an involuntary interruption of the training program because of injuries. Exercise-induced amenorrhea is associated with a reduced bone mass in most of the regions studied, some have found that the most stressed bones are most severely deficient [4], others have found a general effect on the skeleton [5]. In amenorrheic endurance athletes the bone deficit occurs preferentially in vertebral bone [6–8], which is in accordance with the theory that trabecular bone reacts more rapidly to endocrine changes than cortical bone. The frequency of stress fractures is increased both in the athlete with amenorrhea [7] and other menstrual abnormalities [9], and in amenorrheic dancers a high frequency of scoliosis has been described [10]. When amenorrheic and eumeorrheic athletes and nonexercising controls are compared, the general results indicate that the estrogen deficiency state has a more severe impact on the skeleton than exercise, but that exercise may offer some protection on the bones both in the estrogen deficient and estrogen replete women [6, 7, 11].

There is concern about the reversibility of the bone loss associated with amenorrhea. Drinkwater et al. [12] followed seven former amenorrheic athletes who regained menses and found an increase in spinal density after 1 year, but the value in the control group was not reached within the study period. There seems to be a relationship between earlier menstrual history and bone mass, and if the amenorrheic condition has persisted for some years the bone deficit is probably permanent [8]. Oral contraceptives may offer some protection [9], and although we have no long-term data to support the concept, it seems reasonable to supplement the amenorrheic woman with estrogen to prevent her from entering menopause with a low bone mass and an increased fracture risk.

Epidemiological Studies

When bone mass is compared in eumenorrheic young athletic women and nonexercising controls, most studies have found increased bone mass especially in the most stressed parts of the skeleton in the athletic group.

The results are, however, somewhat inconsistent and Buchanan et al. [13] found no difference in trabecular density in a group of women performing endurance sports activities for at least 5 years compared to a control group. Increased bone mass has been described both in athletes performing aerobic and endurance activities but the majority of studies indicate that muscle-building activities are necessary to increase spinal bone density.

After the menopause, both increased [14] and normal [15] spinal density have been found in runners compared to controls. Nelson et al. [16] measured bone density in endurance-trained postmenopausal women and found only small differences in a few of several measured regions. In postmenopausal women a strong correlation has been found between bone density and the amount of exercise up to 300 min per week, but a low density on those exercising more, suggesting that extremely vigorous exercise may be detrimental to bone density in individuals after age 50 [17].

In the nonathletic population interrelations have been found between general fitness, local muscle strength, historical physical activity and bone mass at different sites. A weak relationship has been described between aerobic fitness measured as the maximal oxygen uptake during exercise test, and bone mass in the spine, radius and femur in combined groups of pre- and postmenopausal women [14, 18], but disappeared when the two groups were considered separately. In a recent large study of 300 premenopausal women aged 20–39 years, Mazess and Barden [19] assessed bone density in the spine, femur, forearm and humerus and quantitated activity by accelerators and pedometers worn by all participants for 48 h, and found no relationship between physical activity and bone mass at any site and furthermore found no relationship between activity and rates of bone loss calculated from repeated measurements during 2 years.

These cross-sectional results must be interpreted with caution because of the possibility of selection bias. Women being eumenorrheic in spite of competitive intensive training might have genetic or other characteristics not accounted for and may be able to perform elite athletics because of a high bone mass.

Intervention Studies

Some of the drawbacks with possible selection bias in epidemiological studies are overcome in intervention trials, but new problems may develop. In the vast majority of intervention studies the participants are not randomized. It can naturally be difficult to find participants who volunteer to accept randomization to such different groups as no intervention and intensive training three times a week for several months. However, even in studies where the women have selected treatment according to their preference, the drop-out rates vary between 25 and 33%. In judging the results of intervention studies it is important to know details about the training program and the methods of measuring changes in bone. Most, but not all studies give a thorough description of the training program with details of the type, frequency and intensity including the necessary data on compliance, and in some, active participation is proved by inclusion of data showing increased fitness or strength. The methods of bone measurements have random variation, and methods using radioactive sources may also have systematic variation due to age of source that is not completely corrected for. Both cross-sectional and especially longitudinal bone studies therefore require not only appropriate control groups but also control groups that are measured simultaneously with the active participants. Both photonabsorptiometry and computerized tomography are methods sensitive to changes in body composition. Intensive training decreases fat mass and increases lean body mass. A high fat percent underestimates measured bone mass and a conversion of fat to lean tissue may give false high values of bone mass. Although most methods have programs for correction of variations in soft tissue composition, the effect of increased lean to fat ratio might not be completely eliminated.

The results of intervention in premenopausal women are conflicting. Gleeson et al. [20] studied the effect of weight training 3 times a week in 47 eumenorrheic women and found an increase in lumbar spine density measured by DPA of 0.8% after 1 year compared to a reduction of 0.5% in 44 nonactive controls. The changes in spinal bone were not significant but with a paired t test a difference between the two groups was found, no change was observed in os calcis. Rockwell et al. [21], on the other hand, described a 4% decrease in spinal density measured by quantitative digital radiography during a 9-month weight-training program that included axial loading [21]. No change of spinal bone occurred in the control group, and the femoral bone mass was unchanged in both groups. In these two studies on premenopausal women the diet was supplemented with 500 mg of calcium and in the study of Gleeson et al. [20] some were taking oral contraceptives.

We have more data on the effects of training in the postmenopausal women. In 1978, Aloia et al. [22] described that a 1-year mainly aerobic training program resulted in a difference in total body calcium between 9 active women and 9 controls but no difference in forearm bone mass was noted. In a short study of 6 months in 73 early postmenopausal women White et al. [23] found the same decline in forearm bone mass of 1.6–1.7% in a walking group and controls, while the loss of 0.8% in women performing dancing was not significant. Nelson et al. [24] have also evaluated the effects of walking in this age group and found an increase of spinal density measured with single energy CT of 0.5% in the active group compared to a decline of 7% in the control group, but no changes in the femur, spine or radius measured by SPA and DPA and no change in total body calcium measured by neutron activation. In a population aged 57–83 years Rikli and McManis [25] found that both aerobic training and training supplemented with weight bearing exercises resulted in an increase of forearm bone mass of 1.3% compared to a loss of 2.5% in controls. The changes were insignificant but the final value was higher in the training group than in the control group. In the only randomized study Chow et al. [26] found almost similar effects of aerobic and aerobic plus strengthening exercise on calcium bone index measured by NA with higher values after 1 year compared to controls but no significant changes were noted within the active groups [26]. These short-term studies thus indicate that training does affect the rate of postmenopausal bone loss, but do not agree on which type of exercise gives the best results or where in the skeleton changes occur. Intensive training can increase muscle mass in 1–2 months, but the remodelling cycle of bone tissue has a duration of at least 4–6 months. To ensure that a new steady state is reached, studies on bone changes must have a duration of at least 1 year and preferably longer.

Smith et al. [27] studied the effect of gradually changing training on bone mass in the radius, ulna and humerus in a combined group of pre- and postmenopausal women during 3–4 years. A decrease in bone mass was observed during the first year followed by a gain during the next 2 years. Unfortunately, the control group was followed only during the first 2 years of the study and the peculiar course of bone changes indicated methodological problems. In a later paper [28] the data were corrected for errors due to equipment malfunction and extended to cover 4 years. The general results were that both exercising and nonexercising women lose bone but the decline is smaller in the exercising women at most measuring sites. In the analysis some data points were omitted because of the equipment problems and the rates of loss in premenopausal women was larger than that found in most other studies. In a vigorous weight-bearing training program including stair climbing and jogging three times a week, Dalsky et al. [29] found a gain in spinal bone of 6.1% after 22 months compared to a reduction of 1.1% in the control group. All participants received a daily calcium supplementation of 1,500 mg and some received estrogen replacement therapy. A reevaluation of spinal bone mass 13 months after cessation of training showed no change compared to baseline values, suggesting that continued mechanical loading is necessary to achieve a permanent effect on bone.

In the older population the study of Smith et al. [30] indicated that the bones of nursing home residents can benefit from exercise and some studies on osteoporotics have arrived at the same conclusion [31].

In conclusion: The available data suggest a beneficial effect of physical training on the postmenopausal bone loss, but indicate that a continued effect demands maintenance of the training intensity and that training cannot reverse the bone loss associated with estrogen deficiency. When the menopause-related changes are omitted, there is a relationship between lean body mass and bone mass in both men and women. It is possible that the positive effects of exercise on bones are related to an increased muscle mass. There is no conclusive evidence of a positive effect of training on premenopausal bones and too intensive exercise programs in the young female can cause severe bone deficiencies due to menstrual disturbances.

Bone Mass and Nutrition

In the discussion about the role of nutrition on osteoporosis both the total energy intake, the intake of proteins and the intake of nutrients such as calcium, magnesium, phosphorus, vitamin D and fibers have been suggested as important factors. The intakes of these nutrients are not independent. In western countries for example about two-thirds of the calcium intake comes from dairy products and a high calcium intake is therefore often related to a high intake of vitamin D and phosphorus. The subject that has drawn the most attention, and has been debated most intensively and emotionally, is the role of calcium on bone loss and the development of osteoporotic fractures. Calcium ingestion during childhood and adolescence may have an important impact on peak adult bone mass, but up until now our knowledge about the regulation of bone metabolism during this important time of life is sparse. We have both cross-sectional and longitudinal studies that favor a beneficial effect of calcium on the adult skeleton while others find no relationship between dietary calcium and bone mass and rate of bone loss. Some interventional studies have shown a retardation of postmenopausal bone loss, but others suggest that calcium has no or a very small effect in selected parts of the skeleton. Three recent reviews furthermore came to different conclusions. Kanis and Passmore [32, 33] concluded that 'the evidence that supplemental calcium increases peak adult bone mass or decreases the incidence of fractures in elderly people is not convincing'. Nordin and Heaney [34] interpreted the available publications differently and found 'that the evidence taken as a whole points to an important role for calcium in the genesis and management of postmenopausal osteoporosis'. The authors' recommendations regarding postmenopausal calcium supplementation varied accordingly. In a meta-analysis of 37 published reports representing 49 studies, Cumming [35] concluded that the available data on calcium supplementation in tablet forms suggests 'that a calcium supplement of around 1000 mg/day in early postmenopausal women can prevent the loss of just under 1% of bone mass per year at all bone sites studied except the vertebrae'. During the last year additional important papers have been published and must be included in the discussion.

Recent Studies on Calcium and Bones

In a cohort of perimenopausal women, Slemenda et al. [36] studied the influence of risk factors on bone mass and found no significant influence of dietary calcium on bone mass in radius, lumbar spine or hip, but a small subgroup with a low radial bone mass were characterized by short stature, low body weight, low calcium intake and were smokers. In Mazess and Barden's [19] study on premenopausal women, no clear relation was found between calcium ingestion and bone mass in the spine, femur, humerus and radius or the rate of change in these regions. Stratification of the women into quartiles according to their calcium ingestion showed a slightly lower bone density at all sites in those consuming less than 666 mg of calcium daily. With multiple regression analysis calcium was not a significant predictor of bone mass at any site. Baran et al. [37] conducted a 3-year randomized study where 20 women increased their dietary calcium by an average of 600 mg to a total of just under 1,600 mg/day primarily by dairy products, while 17 controls continued their baseline diets [37]. After 18 months there was no difference in vertebral bone density, but after 3 years the rates of bone density loss was significantly different in the two groups. The dietary supplemented group showed no significant bone loss in contrast to a loss of 1% per year in the control group, leading to a greater bone density in the 'treated group' after 30 and 36 months. In an 8-year follow-up study on 60 postmenopausal women, van Beresteijn et al. [38] stratified women into three groups according to their habitual calcium ingestion and found a continuous and similar rate of radial bone loss in all three groups. From this study subsamples with the highest and lowest calcium intakes and rates of forearm bone loss were selected for further analysis [39] and no relationship was found between habitual calcium intake and bone mass in the lumbar spine, femoral neck or spinal deformity index. In a 1-year study, Nelson et al. [24] evaluated the effect of walking and milk supplementation corresponding to 831 mg/day in 36 postmenopausal women. The part of the study that dealt with calcium supplementation was randomized and blinded. In women consuming high dietary calcium the femoral bone density increased by 2.0% while the loss in the control group was 1.1%, no difference was observed in lumbar spine, distal radius or total body. Finally, Dawson-Hughes et al. [40] conducted a randomized trail of two different calcium sources on changes in vertebral, femoral and spinal bone in postmenopausal women stratified according to calcium intake. No effect of calcium was observed in early postmenopausal women, but calcium supplementation decreased bone loss in women who had passed the menopause more than 5 years earlier. This effect was, however, only seen in women with a habitual calcium intake of less than 400 mg/day and not in those with a baseline intake of 400–650 mg/day.

In conclusion: The results from longitudinal observational studies on the effect of calcium supplementation on postmenopausal bone loss are conflicting and there is no conclusive evidence of a direct relationship between calcium ingestion and bone mass in other age groups. Compared with the remaining literature the most recent studies indicate, however, that there is a threshold value of calcium intake below which bone loss increases, and that women with the lowest intake are those most likely to benefit from calcium supplementation. Variations in habitual calcium intake may explain some of the conflicting results from earlier intervention trials. There is agreement that estrogen deficiency has a more severe impact on bones than calcium, and calcium supplementation alone cannot prevent the initial, rapid postmenopausal loss of predominately trabecular bone. The role of calcium on bone loss and fractures is not yet settled and in spite of the abundance of literature on the topic, controlled, randomized trials considering menopausal duration, variations in bone mass and habitual calcium intake and different calcium sources are still warranted.

References

1 Cann CE, Martin MC, Genant HK, et al: Decreased spinal mineral content in amenorrheic women. JAMA 1984;251:626–629.
2 Davies MC, Hall ML, Jacobs HS: Bone mineral loss in young women with amenorrhoea. Br Med J 1990;301:790–793.
3 Prior JC, Vigna YM, Schechter MT, et al: Spinal bone loss and ovulatory disturbances. N Engl J Med 1990;323:1221–1227.
4 Warren MP, Brooks-Gunn J, Fox RP, et al: Lack of bone accretion and amenorrhea: Evidence for a relative osteopenia in weight-bearing bones. J Clin Endocrinol Metab 1991;72:847–853.
5 Lindberg JS, Fears WB, Hunt MM, et al: Exercise-induced amenorrhea and bone density. Ann Intern Med 1984;101:647–648.
6 Drinkwater BL, Nilson K, Chesnut CH, et al: Bone mineral content of amenorrheic and eumenorrheic athletes. N Engl J Med 1984;311:277–281.
7 Marcus R, Cann C, Madvig P, et al: Menstrual function and bone mass in elite women distance runners. Endocrine and metabolic features. Ann Intern Med 1985; 102:158–163.
8 Drinkwater BL, Bruemner B, Chesnut CH: Menstrual history as a determinant of current bone density in young athletes. JAMA 1990;263:545–548.
9 Barrow GW, Saha S: Menstrual irregularity and stress fractures in collegiate female distance runners. Am J Sports Med 1988;16:209–216.
10 Warren MP, Brooks-Gunn J, Hamilton LH, et al: Scoliosis and fractures in young ballet dancers. Relation to delayed menarche and secondary amenorrhea. N Engl J Med 1986;314:1348–1353.
11 Wolman RL, Clark P, McNally E, et al: Menstrual state and exercise as determinants of spinal trabecular bone density in female athletes. Br Med J 1990;301:516–518.
12 Drinkwater BL, Nilson K, Ott S, et al: Bone mineral density after resumption of menses in amenorrheic athletes. JAMA 1986;256:380–382.
13 Buchanan JR, Myers C, Lloyd T, et al: Determinants of peak trabecular bone density in women: The role of androgens, estrogen, and exercise. J Bone Mineral Res 1988; 3:673–680.
14 Lane NE, Bloch DA, Jones HH, et al: Long-distance running, bone density, and osteoarthritis. JAMA 1986;255:1147–1151.
15 Kirk S, Sharp CF, Elbaum N, et al: Effect of long-distance running on bone mass in women. J Bone Miner Res 1989;4:515–522.
16 Nelson ME, Meredith CN, Dawson-Hughes B, et al: Hormone and bone mineral status in endurance-trained and sedentary postmenopausal women. J Clin Endocrinol Metab 1988;66:927–933.
17 Michel BA, Bloch DA, Fries JF: Weight-bearing exercise, overexercise, and lumbar bone density over age 50 years. Arch Intern Med 1989;149:2325–2329.

18 Pocock NA, Eisman JA, Yeates MG, et al: Physical fitness is a major determinant of femoral neck and lumbar spine bone mineral density. J Clin Invest 1986;78:618–621.
19 Mazess RB, Barden HS: Bone density in premenopausal women: Effects of age, dietary intake, physical activity, smoking, and birth-control pills. Am J Clin Nutr 1991;53:132–142.
20 Gleeson PB, Protas EJ, LeBlanc AD, et al: Effects of weight lifting on bone mineral density in premenopausal women. J Bone Mineral Res 1990;5:153–158.
21 Rockwell JC, Sorensen AM, Baker S, et al: Weight training decreases vertebral bone density in premenopausal women: A prospective study. J Clin Endocrinol Metab 1990;71:988–993.
22 Aloia JF, Cohn SH, Ostuni JA, et al: Prevention of involutional bone loss by exercise. Ann Intern Med 1978;89:356–358.
23 White MK, Martin RB, Yeater RA, et al: The effects of exercise on the bones of postmenopausal women. Int Orthop 1984;7:209–214.
24 Nelson ME, Fisher EC, Dilmanian FA, et al: A 1-y walking program and increased dietary calcium in postmenopausal women: Effects on bone. Am J Clin Nutr 1991; 53:1304–1311.
25 Rikli RE, McManis BG: Effects of exercise on bone mineral content in postmenopausal women. Res Q Exerc Sport 1990;61:243–249.
26 Chow R, Harrison JE, Notarius C: Effect of two randomized programmes on bone mass of healthy postmenopausal women. Br Med J 1987;295:1441–1444.
27 Smith EL, Smith PE, Ensign CJ, et al: Bone involution decrease in exercising middle-aged women. Calcif Tissue Int 1984;36:S129–138.
28 Smith EL, Gilligan C, McAdam M, et al: Deterring bone loss by exercise intervention in premenopausal and postmenopausal women. Calcif Tiss Int 1989;44:312–321.
29 Dalsky GP, Stocke KS, Ehsani AA, et al: Weight-bearing exercise training and lumbar bone mineral content in postmenopausal women. Ann Intern Med 1988;108: 824–828.
30 Smith EL, Reddan W, Smith PE: Physical activity and calcium modalities for bone mineral increase in aged women. Med Sci Sports Exerc 1981;13:60–64.
31 Simkin A, Ayalon J, Leichter I: Increased trabecular bone density due to bone-loading exercises in postmenopausal osteoporotic women. Calcif Tissue Int 1987;40: 59–63.
32 Kanis JA, Passmore R: Calcium supplementation of the diet-I. Br Med J 1989;298: 137–140.
33 Kanis JA, Passmore R: Calcium supplementation of the diet-II. Br Med J 1989;298: 205–208.
34 Nordin BEC, Heaney RP: Calcium supplementation of the diet: Justified by present evidence. Br Med J 1990;300:1056–1060.
35 Cumming RG: Calcium intake and bone mass: A quantitative review of the evidence. Calcif Tissue Int 1990;47:194–201.
36 Slemenda CW, Hui SL, Longcope C, et al: Predictors of bone mass in perimenopausal women. A prospective study using photon absorptiometry. Ann Intern Med 1990;112:96–101.

37 Baran D, Sorensen A, Grimes J, et al: Dietary modification with dairy products for preventing vertebral bone loss in premenopausal women: A three-year prospective study. J Clin Endocrinol Metab 1989;70:264–270.
38 van Beresteijn ECH, van't Hof MA, de Waard H, et al: Relation of axial bone mass to habitual dietary calcium intake and to cortical bone loss in healthy early postmenopausal women. Bone 1990;11:7–13.
39 van Beresteijn ECH, van't Hof MA, Schaafsma G, et al: Habitual dietary calcium intake and cortical bone loss in perimenopausal women: A longitudinal study. Calcif Tissue Int 1990;47:338–344.
40 Dawson-Hughes B, Dallal GE, Krall EA, et al: A controlled trial of the effect of calcium supplementation on bone density in postmenopausal women. N Engl J Med 1990;323:878–883.

Lisbeth Nilas, PhD, Department of Clinical Chemistry, Glostrup Hospital, DK–2600 Glostrup (Denmark)

Panel VI
New Concepts on Nutrition, Fitness and RDAs

Simopoulos AP (ed): Nutrition and Fitness in Health and Disease.
World Rev Nutr Diet. Basel, Karger, 1993, vol 72, pp 114–127

In situ Kinetics and Ascorbic Acid Requirements

Mark Levine[a], *Cathy C. Cantilena*[b], *Kuldeep R. Dhariwal*[a]

[a] Laboratory of Cell Biology and Genetics, National Institute of Diabetes and Digestive and Kidney Diseases, and [b] Department of Transfusion Medicine, Warren Grant Magnuson Clinical Center, National Institutes of Health, Bethesda, Md., USA

Introduction

Ascorbic acid (vitamin C) is required for human health [1], but the optimal amount is unknown [2]. Rather than providing optimal ingestion, the Recommended Dietary Allowance (RDA) has a different basis: preventing deficiency symptoms, reaching the threshold for urinary excretion, and maintaining a target body pool size [1]. Deficiency symptoms can be prevented with as little as 10–12 mg ascorbic acid daily [3–5]. The US RDA of 60 mg provides a margin of safety against deficiency [1]. The threshold for urinary excretion was thought to occur when ingestion was 60 mg daily [5–7]. Once vitamin appears in urine, additional ingestion is considered unnecessary, and even wasteful [1]. The RDA target body pool size of 1,500 mg is reached just as urinary excretion occurs.

By these criteria, the RDA for vitamin C from many countries prevents deficiency in populations. However, it is of fundamental importance to recognize that preventing deficiency may not be the same as providing an optimal amount [2].

There are several specific problems with principles of the RDA. If vitamin C had a narrow therapeutic window, using deficiency prevention as an endpoint is proper. Despite misconceptions, vitamin C is remarkably nontoxic [2, 8–11] (table 1). Although kidney stones, destruction of vitamin B_{12} rebound scurvy (conditioning), and hemolysis have all been suggested to be caused by vitamin C, the evidence does not support the claims

Table 1. Adverse effects of vitamin C ingestion in humans

Vitamin C toxicity
Diarrhea: >3–4 g once orally
Iron absorption: hemochromatosis, thalassemia major, sideroblastic anemia
False negatives for occult blood in stool
??? Oxalate hypersecretion and kidney stones; possible for doses greater than 4 g daily
??? Hyperuricosuria: intravenous doses greater than 2 g once
??? Hyperoxalemia in dialysis patients
Misconceptions of vitamin C toxicity
Rebound scurvy (conditioning)
Hemolysis
Mutagenesis
Venous stasis
Destruction of vitamin B_{12} in food

(table 1). Therefore, it is inappropriate to use prevention of deficiency as an endpoint because of toxicity concerns, since these concerns are unwarranted in healthy people except in special cases (table 1). Indeed, by consuming a diet rich in fruits and vegetables we can ingest approximately 7 times the RDA, and our paleolithic forbearers were estimated to eat nearly 7-fold the RDA for ascorbic acid [12].

Urinary excretion of vitamin C has been taken to indicate saturation of body stores [1, 5–7, 13]. It is not clear from the data, though, that saturation truly occurred at the urinary threshold. For some substances such as glucose, urinary excretion indicates pathology as well as saturation. For other substances such as magnesium, potassium, and even sodium, urinary excretion does not correlate with body stores. It is unknown whether urinary excretion indicates saturation of ascorbic acid. The urinary excretion data themselves may be incorrect due to nonspecific assay techniques [14]. Since the assays overestimate ascorbic acid at low concentrations, the reported threshold may be too low. In addition, the volunteers used for some urinary excretion experiments were outpatients instructed to adhere to diets. Variability in the data may indicate a lack of dietary compliance. Unfortunately, dietary intake data alone can be notoriously inaccurate [15]. If the volunteers ingested more ascorbic acid than believed, the ingestion calculated to produce urinary excretion will again be artificially too low.

The RDA is also based on an ideal body pool size. This body pool size is based in part on the urinary excretion studies above, which may be flawed. The body pool calculations are based on pharmacokinetic assumptions of vitamin C absorption and compartmentalization [4–7]. The calculations may be incorrect due to assay nonspecificity, a narrow dose range, lack of bioavailability data, uncertainty about true ingestion in the volunteers, and undocumented purity of radiolabelled ascorbic acid given to patients and in the samples obtained from them. Other assumptions on which the pharmacokinetics are based, such as constant fractional excretion and existence of three compartments, may also be incorrect.

For all of these reasons, the RDA may not represent optimal vitamin C ingestion. How, then, has optimal vitamin C ingestion been measured? Simply stated, it has not been clear what measurement indicates optimal vitamin C ingestion. Some approaches have their roots in reports of vitamin C depletion in tissues of experimentally infected animals and vitamin C inactivation of viruses [16, 17]; such data were one basis of testing whether vitamin C could prevent colds [18, 19]. Other approaches are based on the experimental observations of vitamin C depletion in adrenal glands mediated by ACTH [20, 21]; these data were interpreted to indicate vitamin C involvement in stress [22]. The consequences have been to use heat stress, cold stress, athletic endurance, or resistance to infection as assays to measure optimal vitamin C ingestion. As might be expected, these approaches have not succeeded, except to generate controversy and even derision.

In situ Kinetics: Biochemical Component

How can optimal requirements for vitamin C, or for any vitamin, be determined? The missing component from all of these approaches is to relate vitamin function to vitamin amount, or vitamin concentration. We need to know, simply stated, 'How much does what?' Vitamin C is an electron donor for maximal activity of at least 8 isolated enzymes, and may be a reducing agent for other reactions (table 2) [23–42]. To understand optimal requirements, we need to learn how different concentrations of vitamin C regulate these reactions, enzymatic and nonenzymatic. The action of the vitamin must be studied in situ, meaning in cells, organelles, tissues, animals, and eventually humans. Study of the reactions in situ is essential because the reactions for isolated proteins or isolated reactions may be different, especially for a reducing agent like ascorbic acid. Optimal requirements will come from determining curves of vitamin concen-

Table 2. Biochemical function of ascorbic acid in enzymatic and chemical reactions

Enzymatic function	
Proline hydroxylase (EC 1.14.11.2)	collagen synthesis
Procollagen-proline 2-oxoglutarate 3-dioxygenase (EC 1.14.11.7)	collagen synthesis
Lysine hydroxylase (EC 1.14.11.4)	collagen synthesis
Gamma-butyrobetaine, 2-oxoglutarate 4-dioxygenase (EC 1.14.11.1)	carnitine synthesis
Trimethyllysine-2-oxoglutarate dioxygenase (EC 1.14.11.8)	carnitine synthesis
Dopamine beta-monooxygenase (EC 1.14.17.3)	catecholamine synthesis
Peptidyl glycine alpha-amidating monooxygenase (EC 1.14.17.3)	peptide amidation
4-Hydroxyphenylpyruvate dioxygenase (EC 1.13.11.27)	tyrosine metabolism
Chemical reactions	
?Prevention of LDL oxidation	
?Quenching of reactive oxidants	
Iron absorption	
Function unknown: tissue contains high concentrations	
Host defense	
Neutrophils, monocytes, B lymphocytes, T lymphocytes, platelets	
Endocrine	
Adrenal cortex, testes, ovaries, pancreas	
Vision	
Lens	

tration versus its function in situ, for many functions depending on the vitamin. Optimal may be that concentration which causes reactions to achieve V_{max}, yet without toxicity. For optimal to be equivalent to maximal rate, the measured rate for at least one reaction system in situ should be V_{max}, with endogenous concentration of vitamin. These principles are based on determining reaction kinetics in situ, and are therefore called in situ kinetics.

In situ kinetics has 2 general components. The biochemical component is to determine how vitamin C-dependent reactions are regulated by vitamin C concentration, and to be able to measure both the vitamin and the reaction in human tissue. The biochemical portion of in situ kinetics was verified for the first time using norepinephrine synthesis in animal tissue [44–51]. These studies are the first demonstration of in situ kinetics for any vitamin using endogenous substrate and the endogenous vitamin. The concept of in situ kinetics, especially its biochemical basis, has been described in detail elsewhere [2, 52–55]. For many of these studies, animal tissue was used and provided a useful and practical model system. The biochemical principles of in situ kinetics now are being extended to human tissue, where they are most relevant to vitamin requirements.

In situ Kinetics: Clinical Component

The clinical component of in situ kinetics is to determine how different concentrations of vitamin C, which regulate the specific reactions in situ, can be achieved in humans as a function of ingestion. The concentration of vitamin C must be determined not only in the circulation, but in other tissues where vitamin C dependent reactions occur. In the remainder of this article we will concentrate on the clinical component of in situ kinetics.

To learn what concentrations are achieved in relation to dose, several prerequisites should be met. Measurements of vitamin C in plasma and tissues must be accurate. The assay must provide sensitivity, specificity, stability for a substance which usually oxidizes easily, and a means to overcome interfering substances [14]. Such an assay is now available and has already been used to measure ascorbic acid in blood, neutrophils, lymphocytes, and monocytes [14, 40, 41, 47, 49, 53].

It should be understood whether ascorbic acid is found in plasma and tissues as ascorbic acid alone, or whether dehydroascorbic acid can also be detected. There are reports that dehydroascorbic acid in plasma or serum represents from 1 to 20% of total ascorbic acid [56–60]. Using a new sensitive and specific HPLC ascorbic acid assay developed in this laboratory, we were unable to detect dehydroascorbic acid in plasma of normal volunteers (table 3) [47, 49, 53, 54]. These volunteers had as much as a 5-fold range in the concentration of ascorbic acid in plasma. The data indicate that dehydroascorbic acid is $<1\%$ of ascorbic acid in normal plasma. These measurements could not distinguish between no dehydroascorbic acid at all versus dehydroascorbic acid concentrations $<1\%$ of ascorbic acid. While it is possible that plasma contains these very small amounts of dehydroascorbic acid, it cannot be detected with the best available assays. A more likely explanation is that dehydroascorbic acid is not present under

Table 3. Ascorbic acid, dehydroascorbic acid, and ascorbic acid protein binding in plasma of normal men and women

Subject	Ascorbic acid	Ascorbic acid + dehydroascorbic acid	Ascorbic acid	
			retentate	filtrate
Women				
1	85.0±0.3	88.0±1.0	83.6±0.0	83.0±0.7
2	40.4±1.1	41.8±0.6	39.3±0.6	39.2±0.7
3	68.2±0.2	67.3±0.7	66.2±0.2	65.0±0.3
4	67.6±0.3	68.2±1.2	67.3±0.9	66.1±0.1
5	78.9±1.3	76.5±1.3	78.1±2.3	73.7±0.5
Men				
1	74.1±0.8	75.6±0.7	75.1±7.2	75.6±1.9
2	22.6±0.6	22.5±1.5	22.2±0.1	21.8±0.1
3	61.3±0.1	60.5±0.9	60.8±0.3	60.0±0.3
4	99.6±0.7	99.7±1.0	99.9±1.5	96.2±1.8
5	20.3±0.1	19.3±0.1	20.1±0.8	19.2±0.9

Since the values in the first and second columns are nearly the same, dehydroascorbic acid is not present. The possibility of protein binding of ascorbic acid was investigated; results are in the third and fourth columns.
Freshly isolated plasma was subjected to centrifugal ultrafiltration for 30 min. If ascorbic acid were protein bound, the concentration in the retentate would be higher than in the filtrate. Since the concentrations in columns 3 and 4 are virtually identical, ascorbic acid is free and not protein bound. The measurements were performed on a total of 20 volunteers for plasma and serum with identical results. Ascorbic acid and dehydroascorbic acid were measured using HPLC with coulometric electrochemical detection. [Data are from references 53 and 54; see refs 47, 49, 53, 54 for experimental details.]

normal conditions. Previous reports of much higher concentrations of dehydroascorbic acid in blood are probably a result of insensitive assay techniques, instability of ascorbic acid in plasma, and inadvertent oxidation to dehydroascorbic acid during the assay procedures [14, 53]. The data indicate that for a dose-response curve in normal people, ascorbic acid is the substance which should be measured.

Another prerequisite to performing an ingestion study in humans is to determine whether ascorbic acid is bound or free. Protein binding may substantially affect subsequent pharmacokinetic calculations. We found that ascorbic acid was not protein bound in 20 normal volunteers, and is free in the circulation (table 3) [53, 54].

Since ascorbic acid can be measured accurately in plasma, the form of ascorbic acid in plasma is ascorbic acid alone, and the vitamin is not protein bound, an ingestion study can be designed. The goal is to determine how ingestion over a wide range regulates plasma and tissue concentration. Surprisingly, such a study has never been performed; it is unknown how a wide range of ingestion regulates plasma concentration. Ingestion studies were performed over a narrow range, or ingestion was studied at either low or high doses with little or no midpoint data [3–7, 61–68]. Most of these studies were performed using less specific assays or without controlling for ascorbic acid oxidation. In many cases, vitamin C intake was estimated by questionnaire and not by controlling intake.

Why is a dose ingestion curve necessary? The concentrations which regulate ascorbic acid transport to essential tissues are under investigation [40, 41, 69]. The K_m of ascorbic acid transport in neutrophils is 2–5 μM [40], and for fibroblasts and lymphocytes is approximately 10 μM [manuscript in preparation]. To learn about optimal requirements, it should be known how ingestion provides plasma concentrations which will affect transport, and ultimately function. Plasma concentrations may be within the range of K_m for transport, substantially above, or substantially below. These possibilities are displayed in figure 1. Each outcome has a different implication for vitamin C requirements. For example, if nearly every ingestion amount provides a plasma concentration substantially above K_m, then the RDA may be correct, or even an overestimate (curve A, fig. 1). Alternatively, if there is a steep ingestion curve with a plateau substantially above K_m for cellular transport, ideal ingestion for a nontoxic vitamin would be at this plateau and not on the steep portion of the curve. If the RDA was on the steep portion, small differences in ingestion would cause large changes in internal concentrations, affecting the amount of vitamin available for specific intracellular reactions (see curve B, fig. 1). Still another possibility is that there is a more gradual rise in plasma concentrations with respect to ingestion. In this case, plasma vitamin concentrations would be in the same range as K_m of transport and/or function over a wider amount of ingestion (curve C, fig. 1).

An ingestion curve is valuable not just for plasma but also for accessible tissues which contain vitamin C, such as neutrophils, platelets, monocytes, lymphocytes, and semen [40, 41, 70–72]. It should be possible to determine how these tissues saturate in comparison to plasma. Urinary excretion could also be determined with respect to ingestion, to test whether saturation has a relationship to excretion of ascorbic acid.

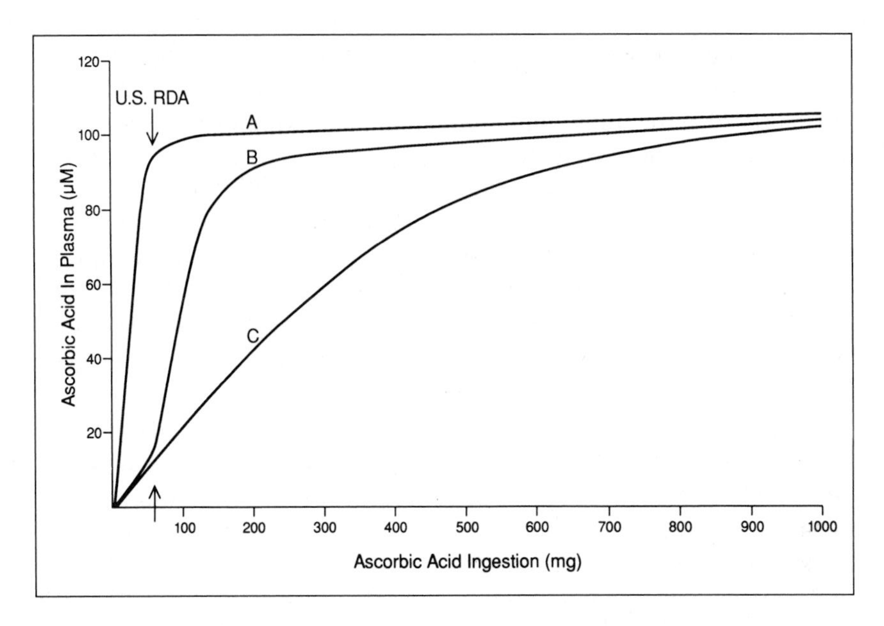

Fig. 1. Theoretical curves of ascorbic acid concentration in plasma as a function of ingestion. Curves A, B, and C represent three different possibilities as to how ingestion regulates plasma concentration. The arrows indicate the US RDA for vitamin C. See text for details.

We have designed a study in normal humans to achieve these goals, to learn for the first time how ingestion regulates concentration. Normal men and women volunteers will be hospitalized for 4 months. To control food intake, only inpatient volunteers will be studied. All food intake is provided on a hospital ward and is strictly monitored daily. For the first 3- to 4-week phase, biochemical deficiency will be achieved without clinical symptoms of scurvy. Volunteers will receive a defined diet containing ≤5 mg daily ascorbic acid. Plasma concentrations will be measured every 3–4 days. A target plasma concentration of 10 μ*M* was selected, because symptoms of scurvy were reported at concentrations ≤10 μ*M* [3–5]. It is very likely that these plasma values were overestimates, due to nonspecificity of the assay especially at lower ascorbic acid concentrations [14]. Other investigators have depleted volunteers to plasma concentrations of ≤5 μ*M*, without symptoms of scurvy [61, 62]. Since body stores will not be completely depleted at a plasma concentration of 10 μ*M*, repletion at lower doses should be possible within 2–3 weeks. Clinical scurvy is to be avoided, so no harm comes to volunteers. If the target plasma concentration were below 5 μ*M*, it is possible that repletion at low doses would take too long, so that the study could not be completed within 4 months, or that higher doses would have to be eliminated.

Once target plasma concentrations are achieved, volunteers will remain on the ascorbic acid-deficient diet for the duration of the study. Vitamin C will be given as a pure substance in 6–7 doses, ranging from 30 to 2,500 mg. At each dose, samples will be taken every 2–3 days until plasma concentration reaches a plateau. When the plateau for each dose is compared, these data will provide the first information as to how a range of ingestion controls plasma concentration.

Bioavailability will be determined at each dose using oral and intravenous ascorbic acid, with measurements of ascorbic acid in urine as well as plasma. Renal clearance of ascorbic acid can be determined using an assay that does not have an artificially evelvated baseline that may have given misleading results about clearance [3–7, 14, 73]. The data should allow us to determine how urinary excretion occurs as a function of ascorbic acid concentration, and whether in fact urinary excretion indicates saturation of body stores. These data will also provide new information to develop a pharmacokinetic model of ascorbic acid in humans.

Plasma ascorbic acid concentrations in humans and animals might be hormonally regulated [56, 74–76]. These data are difficult to interpret due to impure hormone preparations, assay difficulties for ascorbic acid, and confounding variables in animal experiments. Nevertheless, hormonal control of plasma ascorbic acid could have substantial clinical implications. Therefore, at plateau for each dose, vitamin C will be sampled every hour for 24 h to determine whether an endogenous rhythm occurs which could be hormonally mediated. These data will also provide new information about when is the best time to sample ascorbic acid; this is currently not known.

To determine ascorbic acid content in tissues, ascorbic acid will be measured at different ingestion doses in neutrophils, monocytes, lymphocytes, platelets, semen, and perhaps saliva. Since ascorbic acid has been postulated to have an inverse relationship with cholesterol [77, 78], apoproteins [79], triglycerides [77], and uric acid [80], these substances will be measured at plateau of each ascorbic acid dose.

Oxalic acid excretion has been postulated to increase as ascorbic acid ingestion increases, and oxalic acid renal stones were proposed to be caused by ascorbic acid [10]. This is probably incorrect, since some oxalic acid assays are falsely elevated by ascorbic acid [10, 81]. Nevertheless, we will measure oxalic acid excretion at different ascorbic acid doses to determine whether there is a possibility of increased oxalic acid excretion at higher ascorbate doses.

Other clinical parameters which appear in frank scurvy will be monitored. These include gingival health, psychometric profiling, and bleeding time. While it is unlikely that these parameters will be affected, they might reveal effects of low ascorbic acid doses.

One major pitfall to a clinical study of ascorbic acid is its assay. The data indicate that the HPLC coulometric electrochemical detection of ascorbic acid in plasma and tissues is sensitive, specific, reproducible, and provides stability [14, 47, 53]. Another problem is related to maintaining a scorbutic diet for 4 months. Using computer modeling, a palatable diet has been developed to make this study possible. To minimize volunteer boredom, volunteers are part of the normal volunteer program at the National Institutes of Health. Except for 24-hour sampling periods, volunteers have most of their days as free time, which they can use to work in one of the hundreds of participating laboratories in the normal volunteer program.

Conclusion

The optimal amount of ascorbic acid for humans remains unknown. Optimal requirements can be determined by learning how biochemical function is regulated by vitamin concentration, and how these concentrations are achieved in humans. Biochemical evidence indicates that this approach is feasible. Clinical evidence is needed to learn whether ascorbic acid concentrations can be achieved which control biochemical function, and to reveal how ascorbic acid concentrations are regulated by ingestion. For the first time, these clinical studies are possible. In situ kinetics offers a new approach to achieving optimal requirements for vitamin C, and for other vitamins.

References

1 Recommended Dietary Allowances: Subcommittee on the 10th Edition of the RDAs, Food and Nutrition Board, Commission on Life Sciences, National Research Council, ed 10. Washington, Nation Academy Press, 1989, pp 115–124.
2 Levine M: N Engl J Med 1986;314:892–902.

3 Hodges RE, Baker EM, Hood J, Sauberlich HE, March SC: Experimental scurvy in man. Am J Clin Nutr 1969;22:535–548.
4 Hodges RE, Hood J, Canham JE, Sauberlich HE, Baker EM: Clinical manifestations of ascorbic acid deficiency in man. Am J Clin Nutr 1971;24:432–443.
5 Baker EM, Hodges RE, Hood J, Sauberlich HE, March SC, Canham JE: Metabolism of ^{14}C and ^{3}H-labeled *l*-ascorbic acid in human scurvy. Am J Clin Nutr 1971;24: 444–454.
6 Kallner A, Hartman D, Hornig D: Steady-state turnover and body pool of ascorbic acid in man. Am J Clin Nutr 1979;32:530–539.
7 Baker EM, Hodges RE, Hood J, Sauberlich HE, March SC: Metabolism of ascorbic 1-14C acid in experimental human scurvy. Am J Clin Nutr 1969;22:549–558.
8 Stein HB, Hasan A, Fox IH: Ascorbic acid induced uricosuria. Ann Intern Med 1976;84:385–388.
9 Balcke P, Schmidt P, Zazgornik J, Kopsa H, Haubenstock A: Ascorbic acid aggravates secondary hpyeroxalemia in patients on chronic hemodialysis. Ann Intern Med 1984;101:344–346.
10 Piesse JW: Nutritional factors in calcium containing kidney stones with particular emphasis on vitamin C. Int Clin Nutr Rev 1985;5:110–129.
11 Rivers J: Safety of high level vitamin C ingestion. Ann NY Acad Sci 1987;498: 445–453.
12 Eaton SB, Konner M: Paleolithic nutrition. N Engl J Med 1985;312:283–289.
13 Baker EM, Saari JC, Tolbert BM: Ascorbic acid metabolism in man. Am J Clin Nutr 1966;19:371–378.
14 Washko PW, Welch RW, Dhariwal KR, Wang Y, Levine M: Ascorbic acid and dehydroascorbic acid analysis in biological samples. Anal Biochem 1992, in press.
15 Hegsted DM: Defining a nutritious diet: Need for new dietary standards. J Am Coll Nutr 1992;11:241–245.
16 Torrance CC: Diphtherial intoxication and vitamin C content of the suprarenals of guinea pigs. J Biol Chem 1940;132:575–584.
17 Jungleblut CW: Inactivation of poliomyelitis virus by crystalline vitamin C (ascorbic acid). J Exp Med 1935;62:517–521.
18 Cowan DW, Diehl HS, Baker AB: Vitamins for the prevention of colds. JAMA 1942; 120:1268–1271.
19 Truswell AS: Ascorbic acid and the common cold. N Engl J Med 1986;315:709.
20 Sayers G, Sayers MA, Liang T, Long CNH: The effect of pituitary adrenotrophic hormone on the cholesterol and ascorbic acid content of the adrenal of the rat and the guinea pig. Endocrinology 1946;38:1–9.
21 Sayers G, Sayers MA: Regulation of pituitary adrenocorticotrophic activity during the response of the rat to acute stress. Endocrinology 1947;40:265–273.
22 Pirani CL: Relation of vitamin C to adrenocortical function and stress phenomena. Metabolism 1952;1:197–222.
23 Peterkofsky B, Udenfriend S: Enzymatic hydroxylation of proline microsomal polypeptide leading to formation of collagen. Proc Natl Acad Sci USA 1965;53:335–342.
24 Kivirikko KI, Prockop DJ: Enzymatic hydroxylation of proline and lysine in protocollagen. Proc Natl Acad Sci USA 1967;57:782–789.

25 Myllyla R, Kuutti-Savolainen E-R, Kivirikko KI: The role of ascorbate in the prolyl hydroxylase reaction. Biochem Biophys Res Commun 1978;83:441–448.

26 Tryggvason K, Risteli J, Kivirikko KI: Separation of prolyl 3-hydroxylase and 4-hydroxylase activities and the 4-hydroxyproline requirement for synthesis of 3-hydroxyproline. Biochem Biophys Res Commun 1977;76:275–281.

27 Puistola U, Turpeeniniemi-Hujanen TM, Myllyla R, Kivirikko KI: Studies on the lysyl hydrolase reaction: Initial velocity kinetics and related aspects. Biochim Biophys Acta 1980;611:40–50.

28 Lindstedt G, Lindstedt S: Cofactor requirementss of gamma-butyrobetaine hydroxylase from rat liver. J Biol Chem 1970;245:4178–4186.

29 Hulse JD, Ellis Sr, Henderson LM: Carnitine biosynthesis: Beta-hydroxylation of trimethyllysine by an alpha-ketoglutarate-dependent mitochondrial dioxygenase. J Biol Chem 1978;253:1654–1659.

30 Dunn WA, Rettura G, Seifter E, Englard S: Carnitine biosynthesis from gamma-butyrobetaine and from exogenous protein bound 6-N-trimethyl-*L*-lysine by the perfused guinea pig liver: Effect of ascorbate deficiency on the in situ activity of gamma-butyrobetaine hydroxylase. J Biol Chem 1984;259:10764–10770.

31 Friedman S, Kaufman S: 3,4-Dihydroxyphenylethylamine beta-hydroxylase. J Biol Chem 1965;240:4763–4773.

32 La Du BN, Zannoni VG: The role of ascorbic acid in tyrosine metabolism. Ann NY Acad Sci 1961;92:175–191.

33 Stoffers DA, Green CB, Eipper BA: Alternative mRNA splicing generates multiple forms of peptidyl-glycine alpha amidating monooxygenase in rat atrium. Proc Natl Acad Sci USA 1989;86:735–739.

34 Lindblad B, Lindstedt G, Lindstedt S, Rundgren M: Purification and some properties of human 4-hydroxyphenyl-pyruvate dioxygenase. J Biol Chem 1977;252:5073–5084.

35 Jialal I, Vega GL, Grundy SM: Physiologic levels of ascorbate inhibit the oxidative modification of low density lipoprotein. Atherosclerosis 1990;82:185–191.

36 Steinberg D, Parthasarathy S, Carew TE, Khoo JC, Witztum JL: Beyond cholesterol: Modifications of low-density lipoprotein that increase its atherogenicity. N Engl J Med 1989;320:915–923.

37 Frei B, Stocker R, Ames BN: Ascorbate is an outstanding antioxidant in human blood plasma. Proc Natl Acad Sci USA 1989;86:6377–6381.

38 Tannenbaum SR, Wishnok JS: Inhibition of nitrosamine formation by ascorbic acid. Ann NY Acad Sci 1987;498:354–363.

39 Cook JD, Watson SS, Simpson KM, Lipschitz DA, Skikne BS: The effect of high ascorbic acid supplementation on body iron stores. Blood 1984;64:721–726.

40 Washko P, Rotrosen D, Levine M: Ascorbic acid transport and accumulation in human neutrophils. J Biol Chem 1989;264:18996–19002.

41 Bergsten P, Amitai G, Kehrl J, Dhariwal K, Klein H, Levine M: Millimolar concentrations of vitamin C in purified mononuclear leukocytes: Depletion and reaccumulation. J Biol Chem 1990;265:2584–2587.

42 Levine M, Morita K: Ascorbic acid in endocrine systems. Vitam Horm 1985;42: 1–64.

43 Robertson J, Donner AP, Trevithick JR: A possible role for vitamins C and E in cataract prevention. Am J Clin Nutr 1991;53:346S–351S.

44 Levine M, Morita K, Pollard HB: Enhancement of norepinephrine biosynthesis by ascorbic acid in cultured bovine chromaffin cells. J Biol Chem 1985;260:12942–12947.
45 Levine M, Morita K, Heldman E, Pollard HB: Ascorbic acid regulation of norepinephrine biosynthesis in isolated chromaffin granules from bovine adrenal medulla. J Biol Chem 1985;260:15598–15603.
46 Levine M: Ascorbic acid specifically enhances dopamine betamonooxygenase activity in resting and stimulated chromaffin cells. J Biol Chem 1986;261:7347–7356.
47 Washko P, Hartzell WO, Levine M: Ascorbic acid analysis using high performance liquid chromatography with coulometric electrochemical detection. Anal Biochem 1989;181:276–282.
48 Dhariwal KR, Washko P, Hartzell WO, Levine M: Ascorbic acid within chromaffin granules: In situ kinetics of norepinephrine biosynthesis. J Biol Chem 1989;264: 15404–15409.
49 Dhariwal K, Washko PW, Levine M: Determination of dehydroascorbic acid using high performance liquid chromatography with coulometric electrochemical detection. Anal Biochem 1990;189:18–23.
50 Dhariwal K, Shirvan M, Levine M: Ascorbic acid regeneration within chromaffin secretory vesicles: In situ kinetics. J Biol Chem 1991;266:5384–5387.
51 Dhariwal KR, Black CDV, Levine M: Semidehydroascorbic acid as an intermediate in norepinephrine biosynthesis in chromaffin granules. J Biol Chem 1991;266: 12908–12914.
52 Levine M: Vitamin C: Turning over a new leaf. Nutrition 1989;5:428.
53 Dhariwal K, Hartzell W, Levine M: Measurement of ascorbic acid and dehydroascorbic acid in human plasma and serum. Am J Clin Nutr 1991;54:712–716.
54 Levine M, Dhariwal KR, Washko P, Wang Y, Welch R, Bergsten P, Butler EJ: Ascorbic acid and in situ kinetics: A new approach to vitamin requirements. Am J Clin Nutr 1991;54:1157S–1162S.
55 Levine M, Dhariwal KR, Washko P, Welch R, Wang Y-H, Cantilena CC, Yu R: Ascorbic acid and reation kinetics in situ: A new approach to vitamin requirements. J Nutr Sci Vitaminol, in press.
56 Stewart CP, Horn DB, Robson JS: The effect of cortisone and adrenocorticotropic hormone on the dehydroascorbic acid of human plasma. Biochem J 1953;53:254–261.
57 Sabry TH, Fisher KH, Dodds ML: Human utilization of dehydroascorbic acid. J Nutr 1958;64:457–466.
58 Cox BD, Wichelow MJ: The measurement of dehydroascorbic acid and diketogulonic acid in normal and diabetic plasma. Biochem Med 1975;12:183–193.
59 Okamura M: An improved method for determination of *L*-ascorbic acid and *L*-dehydroascorbic acid in blood plasma. Clin Chim Acta 1980;103:259–268.
60 Newill A, Habibzadeh N, Bishop N, Schorah CJ: Plasma levels of vitamin C components in normal and diabetic subjects. Ann Clin Biochem 1984;21:488–490.
61 Jacob RA, Skala JH, Omaye ST: Biochemical indices of human vitamin C status. Am J Clin Nutr 1987;46:818–826.
62 Jacob RA, Pianalto FS, Agee RE: Cellular ascorbate depletion in healthy men. J Nutr 1992;122:1111–1118.

63 Mayersohn M: Ascorbic acid absorption in man – pharmakokinetic implications. Eur J Pharm 1972;19:140–142.
64 Vanderjagt DJ, Garry PJ, Bhagavan HN: Ascorbic acid intake and plasma levels in healthy elderly people. Am J Clin Nutr 1987;46:290–294.
65 Melethil SI, Mason WE, Chiang C-J: Dose dependent absorption and excretion of vitamin C in humans. Int J Pharm 1986;31:83–89.
66 Zetler G, Seidel G, Siegers CP, Iven H: Pharmacokinetics of ascorbic acid in man. Eur J Clin Pharmacol 1976;10:273–282.
67 Blanchard J, Conrad KA, Mead RA, Garry PH: Vitamin C disposition in young and elderly men. Am J Clin Nutr 1990;51:837–845.
68 Blanchard J: Depletion and repletion kinetics of vitamin C in humans. J Nutr 1990; 121:170–176.
69 Butler EJ, Bergsten P, Welch R, Levine M: Ascorbic acic accumulation in normal skin fibroblasts. Am J Clin Nutr 1991;54:1144S–1146S.
70 Berg OC, Huggins C, Hodges CV: Concentration of ascorbic acid and phosphatases in secretion of the male genital tract. Am J Phys 1941;133:82–87.
71 Dawson EB, Harris WA, Rankin WE, Charpentier LA, McGanity WA: Effect of ascorbic on male fertility. Ann NY Acad Sci 1987;498:312–323.
72 Evans RM, Currie L, Campbell A: The distribution of ascorbic acid between various cellular components of blood in normal individuals and its relation to the plasma concentration. Br J Nutr 1982;47:473–482.
73 Friedman GJ, Sherry S, Ralli EP: The mechanism of the excretion of vitamin C by the human kidney at low and normal plasma levels of ascorbic acid. J Clin Invest 1940;19:685–689.
74 Slusher MA, Roberts S: Fate of adrenal ascorbic acid: Relationship to corticosteroid secretion. Endocrinology 1957;61:98–105.
75 Lahiri S, Lloyd BB: The effect of stress and corticotrophin on the concentrations of vitamin C in blood and tissues of the rat. Biochem J 1962;84:478–483.
76 Stefanini M, Rosenthal MC: Hemorrhagic diathesis with ascorbic acid deficiency during administration of anterior pituitary corticotropic hormone (ACTH). Proc Soc Exp Biol Med 1950;75:806–808.
77 Simon JA: Vitamin C and cardiovascular disease: A review. J Am Coll Nutr 1992; 11:107–125.
78 Ginter E: Ascorbic acid in cholesterol metabolism and in detoxification of xenobiotic substances. Nutrition 1989;5:369–374.
79 Rath M, Pauling L: Immunological evidence for the accumulation of lipoprotein(a) in the atherosclerotic lesion of the hypoascorbemic guinea pig. Proc Natl Acad Sci USA 1990;87:9388–9390.
80 Sevanian A, Davies KJA, Hochstein P: Serum urate as an antioxidant for ascorbic acid. Am J Clin Nutr 1991;54:1129S–1134S.
81 Li MG, Madappally MM: Rapid enzymatic determiantion of urinary oxalate. Clin Chem 1989;35:2330–2333.

Mark Levine, MD, Building 8, Room 415, National Institutes of Health,
Bethesda, MD 20892 (USA)

Simopoulos AP (ed): Nutrition and Fitness in Health and Disease.
World Rev Nutr Diet. Basel, Karger, 1993, vol 72, pp 128–147

Are ω3 Fatty Acids Essential Nutrients for Mammals?

Norman Salem, Jr., Glenn R. Ward

Chief, Laboratory of Membrane Biochemistry and Biophysics, DICBR, ADAMHA, NIAAA, 10/3C103, Bethesda, Md., USA

Introduction

In this paper, I would like to discuss the growing evidence that n–3 or, using another name, ω3 fatty acids are essential nutrients for mammals and for man. I will also review the studies performed in my laboratory in which the mechanisms underlying the biological functions of the ω3 fatty acid docosahexaenoic acid have been investigated. For the nonlipid chemists, I would like to first review the nomenclature that is in common use.

In figure 1, four of the most common ω3 fatty acids are depicted. Linolenic (18:3n3) acid is the mother of the longer chain and more unsaturated metabolites shown below it. It may be referred to as 18:3; the first number refers to its chain length and the number after the colon refers to the number of double bonds. The n–3 or ω3, which are used interchangeably, refers to the position of the first double bond when counting from the methyl end. Note that all of these fatty acids have their first double bond three carbons from the methyl end; thus they are ω3 fatty acids. Since chain elongation and desaturation occurs only at the carboxyl end of the molecule in all biological organisms above plants, the family that a fatty acid is in is not subject to change as it is metabolized. Thus, the chain-elongated and desaturated products of 18:3n3, i.e. eicosapentaenoic (20:5n3), docosapentaenoic (22:5n3) and docosahexaenoic (22:6n3) acids, remain ω3 fatty acids.

Various ω3 fatty acids are concentrated in different organisms and tissues in the food chain. The 18:3n3 is found at high levels in many ter-

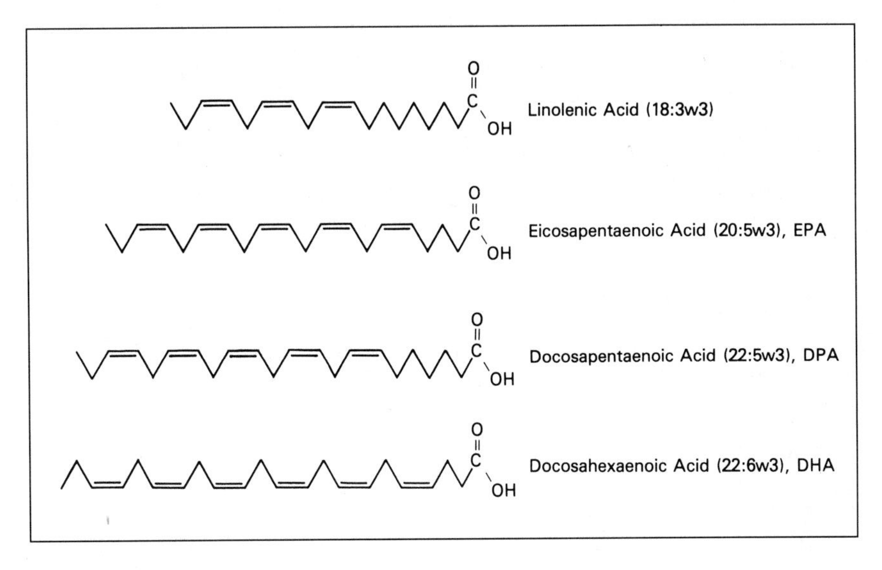

Fig. 1. Structure of the ω3 fatty acids.

restrial and aquatic plants where it is biosynthesized (table 1). However, few terrestrial plants contain longer chain ω3 fatty acids. Aquatic plants often contain high levels of the 20- and 22-carbon ω3 fatty acids, especially 20:5n3. All of these fatty acids may be found in a particular species of aquatic flora or fauna. Zooplankton and marine invertebrates generally have less 18:3n3 and more 20:5n3 than the flora that they feed on. Most fishes have quite high levels of both the 20:5n3 and 22:6n3.

All of these fatty acids are also found in animal tissues (table 2). The longer chain polyunsaturates like 22:6n3 are concentrated in the nervous system. It is interesting to note that the 22:6n3 constitutes 90% or more of the brain ω3 fatty acids; the brain is nearly devoid of 18:3 and 20:5 but does contain some 22:5n3. There are interesting metabolic reasons for this that are not very well understood. Neural and retinal cells contain very high levels of 22:6n3 and it is localized mainly in the aminophospholipids, phosphaditylserine (PS) and phosphatidylethanolamine (PE). It is precisely this pool of ω3 lipid and particularly the 18:0, 22:6-PS that is believed to subserve a critical function. Our analysis of the essentiality of these nutrients will be in large part, although not exclusively, one of evaluation of their role in nervous system function. This includes retinal function since the retina is embryologically derived from neural cells.

Table 1. ω3 fatty acids in the food chain [from ref. 2]

	18:3n3	20:5n3	22:5n3	22:6n3
Aquatic flora				
Golden algae	8.0	3.9	0.1	8.6
Dinoflagellate	0.1	7.4	0.6	25.4
Kelp	6.2	9.7	2.2	4.8
Terrestrial plants				
Barley	64.0	–	–	–
Maize	66.0	–	–	–
Moss	65.0	3.0	–	–
Zooplankton				
Euglena (dark grown)	0.6	13.4	4.5	7.0
Copepod	0.3	12.4	0.1	5.9
Marine invertebrates				
Sponge	0.6	3.6	1.7	15.4
Anemone	0.7	27.1	12.0	19.0
Scallop	1.7	16.1	1.2	30.7
Fish				
Cod	0.1	17.6	0.9	37.5
Pilchard	0.9	16.9	2.5	12.9
Tuna, skipjack	1.2	13.2	1.5	17.3

ω3 Fatty Acid Deficiency

One of the most useful approaches to understanding whether a nutrient is essential and what minimal level is required has been the study of its deprivation and the resulting consequences. Indeed, much of our understanding of the importance of ω3 fatty acids have come from studies of deprivation induced by various means. Therefore, a brief review of these findings is in order.

There are now several excellent reviews which discuss various facets of the essentiality of ω3 fatty acids including those by Salem and co-workers [1, 2], Uauy et al. [3] and Innis [4]. These have focused mainly upon brain, retinal and reproductive functions. It does not appear to be a coincidence that these functions are performed by organs where 22:6n3 is highly concentrated.

Table 2. ω3 fatty acids in mammals [from ref. 2]

Tissue	18:3n3	20:5n3	22:5n3	22:6n3
Human gray matter PE	–	–	tr	24.3
Human gray matter PS	–	–	3.3	36.6
Human gray matter PC	–	–	–	3.1
Human white matter PE	–	–	0.5	3.4
Hyaena gray matter PE	–	–	1.5	24.0
Rat whole brain PE	–	–	0.3	23.7
Rat synaptosomal membrane PE	–	–	nr	32.4
Rat retina PE	–	–	1.2	43.9
Bovine rod outer segment TLE	–	–	1.5	50.7
Human sperm PL	–	–	nr	35.2
Human liver PE	0.2	1.6	4.0	7.7
Cat liver PE	1.3	0.9	0.3	22.0
Human brown adipose TLE	0.3	nr	nr	1.5
Rat heart PE	nr	0.5	2.5	23.4
Rat lung PE	nr	nr	3.8	6.1
Rat spleen PE	nr	nr	3.6	6.0
Rat GI tract PE	nr	nr	1.7	5.5
Human plasma PC	nr	1.3	1.1	4.0
Human erythrocyte TLE	nr	0.8	2.6	5.9
Human milk TLE	0.6	0.2	0.2	0.3

Learning has been assessed in a number of studies, predominantly in the rat (table 3). Among the most common findings are deficits in visual discrimination learning following ω3 fatty acid deprivation throughout development [5, 7, 13], and at least one study has reported that ω3 supplementation during gestation and lactation improved non-visually dependent, active avoidance learning in rats [8]. The reader should be aware of possible confounding effects of abnormal visual function due to ω3 deficiency which have been discussed in a recent review [14]. While activity levels themselves have been reported to be unaffected by ω3 deficiency [5, 6], exploratory activity in a novel environment has been reported to be reduced in at least one study [6].

The rate of behavioral development may be affected by ω3 fatty acids. Although one study has reported no effect of ω3 deficiency on reflex development in rats [7] another study has reported delayed eye-opening in

Table 3. The effects of ω3 essential fatty acid deficiency on brain function in mammals

Subjects	Fat source	Effects	Reference No.
Rats	sunflower vs. soybean oil for two generations	improved shock avoidance in soybean (high ω3) group	5
Rats	safflower vs. soybean oil from before conception to 16 weeks	increased exploratory activity in a novel environment in soybean group	6
Rats	safflower vs. soybean oil from before conception to young adulthood	improved Y-maze performance in soybean group	7
Rats	osmotic pump supplementation of ω3 fatty acids throughout gestation and lactation	improved learning of active avoidance task in supplemented group	8
Rhesus monkeys	safflower vs. soybean oil from before conception to 5 years of age	polydipsia in safflower (low ω3) group	9
Rhesus monkeys	safflower vs. soybean oil from before conception to 30 months of age	polydipsia in safflower group	10
	safflower vs. soybean oil from birth to 30 months of age	polydipsia in safflower group	
Mice	safflower vs. polepa throughout pregnancy and lactation	earlier age of eye opening in ω3 pups	11
Rats	safflower vs. perilla oil for two generations	improved brightness discrimination and faster extinction in perilla oil (high ω3) group	12
Rats	safflower vs. perilla oil from before conception to 20 months of age	improved brightness discrimination learning in senescence in perilla oil group	13

deficient mice [11]. A recent report suggested that aging may also be accelerated in deficient animals [13]. Aged rats are known to exhibit reductions in learning ability on a number of tasks, and feeding of perilla oil (rich in 18:3n3) throughout development and adulthood was found to improve performance in senescent rats over that of rats which had been fed safflower oil. On the other hand, since the performance of the rats fed perilla oil was still less than that of their younger counterparts, these results may not reflect resistance to age-related learning deficits but may be due to improved learning ability at all ages compared with that of their safflower-fed counterparts.

Primates have also been studied as possible models of ω3 fatty acid deficiency. The major behavioral alteration to be reported so far has been polydipsia in the form of increased use of drinking spouts in caged ω3-deficient rhesus monkeys. This polydipsia is associated with increased urine output but does not appear to be due to osmotic imbalances, diabetes mellitus, renal malfunctions, or a general increase in consummatory behavior [9, 15]. Furthermore, this effect was seen in monkeys deprived of ω3 fatty acids during either the postnatal or combined pre- and postnatal period [10]: monkeys deprived only during prenatal development exhibited normal drinking behavior.

Little is known of the effects of ω3 fatty acid deficiency in humans due to the rarity of the phenomenon in most populations. One group which may be deficient, however, is made up of premature, very low birthweight (VLBW) human neonates. These infants are often reared on infant formulas, many of which are low in ω3 polyunsaturates, and devoid of the 22-carbon length ω3 fatty acids, during the period in which much of the long-chain ω3 polyunsaturates are deposited in the developing brain. Unfortunately, few studies have evaluated behavioral and intellectual development in this population. A preliminary report described deficits in these infants on tests of cognition such as the Fagan Infantest and the Bayley Mental and Psychomotor Developmental Indices, but could not attribute these effects specifically to ω3 deficiency [16]. Recently, a report appeared detailing a study of children who had been born prematurely and tube-fed rather than breast-fed during early postnatal life [17]. In this study, however, although all infants were tube-fed, each received either commercial infant formula or breast milk provided by the mother. At 7½–8 years of age, the children in the breast milk-fed group exhibited a mean IQ score almost 9 points above the mean of the formula-fed children. Although major socioeconomic variables were controlled for in this study, the authors point out that the IQ differences still could be attributable to differences between the groups in other parental variables, such as educational level, which may be associated with the decision to provide breast milk at birth, rather than to the nutritional composition of the formulas.

At least one case study has been published implicating ω3 deficiency in severe neurological symptoms [18]. In this study, a 6-year-old girl underwent total parenteral nutrition for several months following gastrointestinal surgery, and subsequently developed severe neurological abnormalities including sensory, motor, and visual deficits. As the initial dietary preparation contained a very low linolenate/linoleate ratio, a new diet containing a higher ratio was administered, and the neurological symptoms improved. Can certain neurological disorders in humans be attributable to deficiencies in tissue levels of docosahexaenoic acid (22:6n3)? At this time, it is impos-

Table 4. Neurological disorders in humans associated with ω3 fatty acid deficiency

Disorder	Neurological symptoms	ω3 EFA status	Reference No.
Kinky hair disease	cerebral and cerebellar degeneration beginning within 2 months of birth severe mental retardation	decreased 22:6n3 in PS and PE fractions	19
Multiple sclerosis	demyelination of axons	decreased 22:6n3 in plaques and normal-appearing white matter relative to gray and white matter, respectively, of controls	20
Polyunsaturated fatty acid lipidosis	progressive encephalopathy beginning in infancy	decreased 22:6n3 in PS and PE fractions in cerebral cortex	21
Juvenile neuronal ceroid-lipofuscinosis	central nervous system degeneration seizures and dementia onset before 8 years of age	decreased 22:6n3 in leukocytes smaller decreases in leukocytes of patients' parents greater decreases in cases of more advanced disease	22
Zellweger's and pseudo-Zellweger's syndrome	psychomotor retardation and visual impairment seizures possible usually fatal before 6 months of age	decreased 22:6n3 in brain, liver and kidney in 'pseudo' form, reductions present but less pronounced	23

sible to attribute causality for particular disorders particularly to ω3 deficiencies, but low levels of 22:6n3 have been correlated with neurological disease in a number of cases (table 4). For example, the degeneration of the CNS seen in 'kinky hair disease' [19], and in Zellweger's and pseudo-Zellweger's syndrome [23] was associated with reductions in 22:6n3 without concurrent reductions in long-chain ω6 polyunsaturates. In young patients with neuronal ceroid-lipofuscinosis, the degree of severity of the neurological symptoms has been reported to be correlated with the degree of deficiency of 22:6n3 as measured in leukocytes [22]. Another syndrome exhibiting encephalopathy similar to that seen in ceroid-lipofuscinosis, polyunsaturated fatty acid lipidosis, has been identified and is also associated with reduced 22:6n3 concentrations [21]. Finally, epidemiological research has shown that populations whose diet consists of high ω3 levels exhibit a much lower incidence of multiple sclerosis than do populations which consume lower levels [24], and at least one paper has reported decreases in 22:6n3 in the cerebral cortices of patients with multiple sclerosis [20]. Although these studies cannot prove that 22:6n3 reductions cause these neurological syndromes, they do suggest that changes in ω3 metabolism are associated with certain cases of severe neuropathology.

The importance of the essential fatty acids for retinal function has been recognized since the 1970s when it was reported that polyunsaturate deficiency dramatically reduced the rate of turnover of rod outer segment disc membranes in the rat retina [25]. This reduction was associated with a reduction in amplitude of the electroretinogram (ERG) [26] which was ameliorated in proportion to the percent weight of essential fatty acid supplementation, ω3 supplementation being more effective than ω6 [27]. One study has reported that ω3-deficient rats exhibit improved ERG responding over time, with decreases in both *a* and *b* wave amplitudes at 4 weeks of age, but normal *b* wave amplitude, and only slight reductions in *a* wave amplitude, in adulthood [5].

More recently, studies have reported a correlation between altered retinal function following ω3 deficiency and impaired visual function. Rhesus monkeys deprived of ω3 fatty acids prior to conception, throughout gestation, and during early postnatal development exhibited alterations in retinal functioning in the form of delayed latency of response in both rods and cones as well as impaired recovery of the dark-adaptation ERG response, and these findings were associated with reduced visual acuity as demonstrated on behavioral tasks [28, 29]. Interestingly, the impairments in retinal function were still seen after dietary rehabilitation with long-chain ω3 fatty acids sufficient to produce normal ω3 levels in body tissues, suggesting that these nutrients are required during a sensitive period of development of the retina and/or brain.

Some researchers have focused on the effects of infant formulas on visual function in VLBW human neonates. Infants raised on corn oil-based formula containing very little ω3 fatty acid were found to exibit reduced photoreceptor sensitivity compared to VLBW infants fed breast milk, which contains both short- and long-chain ω3 polyunsaturates. This difference was seen at 36 weeks postconception but not at 57 weeks, suggesting that rod development was delayed rather than permanently damaged by the deficiency [30]. On the other hand, visual evoked potentials (VEP) and visual acuity, as assessed on preferential looking tasks, were impaired at both ages [31], and these deficits were also seen in full-term infants after several weeks of feeding with corn oil-based formulas. When formulas were supplemented with both short and long-term ω3 fatty acids, the

Table 5. The effects of ω3 essential fatty acid deficiency on visual function in mammals

Subjects and age	Fat Source	Effects	Reference No.
VLBW infants	corn oil-based infant formula	reduced rod photoreceptor sensitivity at 36 weeks postconception but not at 57 weeks	30
VLBW and full-term infants	corn oil-based infant formula	reduced visual acuity at 57 weeks postconception	31
Rats 4 weeks to adults	sunflower vs. soybean oil for two generations	reduced amplitude of electroretinogram at 4 and 6 weeks less reduction in adulthood	5
Rhesus monkeys 24 months	safflower vs. corn oil from before conception up to 24 months of age	reduced visual acuity	28
Rhesus monkeys 24 months	safflower vs. corn oil from before conception up to 24 months of age	delayed peak latency of photoreceptor response impaired recovery of dark-adaptation response reduced visual acuity	29
Adult rats	18:2n6 vs. 18:3n3 for 40 days	reduced amplitude of electroretinogram	27

resulting retinal development did not differ from that of breast milk-fed infants, while infants fed only short-chain ω3 fatty acids exhibited retinal functioning intermediate between those fed the corn oil-based formula and those fed breast milk. Studies of ω3 fatty acid deficiency and retinal function are summarized in table 5.

Certain forms of retinal pathology have been associated with alterations in tissue levels of ω3 fatty acids. Retinitis pigmentosa (RP) refers to a class of disorders characterized by progressive visual loss accompanied by retinal degeneration, and which appear to be inherited in most cases. One of these disorders, autosomal-dominant RP, has been associated with reductions in docosahexaenoic acid concentrations in the retina [32], and similar reductions have been observed in cases of RP-like retinal degeneration in poodles [33] and Abyssinian cats [34]. As in the case of the neuropathologies discussed earlier, a causal relationship between the tissue ω3 reductions and degeneration cannot be ascertained at this time.

There is some evidence that ω3 essential fatty acids may play a role in successful reproduction. Epidemiological studies have reported that gestational length, birthweight, and the frequency of induced labor are all increased in certain populations consuming high levels of ω3 fatty acids [35, 36], and a few reports have noted decreased reproductive success as a result of ω3 deficiency in rats [37] and mice [38]. In the animal studies, it was not known whether this mortality is caused by abnormal maternal physiology, pup physiology, or both. Essential fatty acid deficiency is known to adversely affect the development of the female reproductive system [39] and a recent report described a reduced response by the developing uterus in rats to low levels of 17β-estradiol following three generations on an ω3-deficient diet [40].

The role of ω6 essential fatty acids in skin disorders has been recognized since early in this century. However, recent research suggests that ω3 fatty acids may also play a role in the development of inflammatory skin diseases by their action on eicosanoid metabolism. Arachidonic acid (20:4n6), the ω6 source of many of the major mediators of the inflammatory response, competes with eicosapentaenoic acid (EPA), an ω3 fatty acid, for the same enzyme systems. Therefore, if EPA is supplied in sufficient quantities in a source such as fish oil, competitive inhibition of 20:4n6 may occur, leading to the replacement of 20:4n6 metabolites with those of EPA, which are less potent activators of inflammation. A number of studies have tested the effects of ω3 supplementation on psoriasis with mixed results. Some authors have reported a reduction in the severity of clinical symptoms of psoriasis in patients consuming fish oil [41, 42] while a study with better experimental controls, but administering lower levels of EPA, found no improvement [43]. This latter group did, however, report improvement of the severity of atopic dermatitis following fish oil supplementation in a later study [44]. A report of α-linolenic acid deficiency in humans noted that skin atrophy and scaly dermatitis may be a clinical sign of ω3 deficiency [45].

Although ω3 fatty acids appear to be necessary for normal growth in certain species of fish [46, 47], their role in growth in mammals remains unclear. Rats and mice generally have been reported to grow at similar rates to controls following ω3 deficiency for more than one generation, but there are a small number of published reports of ω3-deficient humans which suggest that this series is essential for normal growth. In the most dramatic case, a 7-year-old girl who had failed to gain weight after 1.5 years on an ω3-deficient diet exhibited rapid increases in both weight and length when ω3 fatty acids were added to her diet [48]. Interestingly, long-chain ω3 polyunsaturates, such as those in fish oil, were found to be much more effective in eliciting weight gain than were the shorter chain, 18-carbon ω3 fatty acids.

Ethanol Effects on ω3 Fatty Acid Levels

One possible dietary change which may lead to alteration of brain docosahexaenoic acid concentrations in adults is alcohol abuse [49]. Several studies [50, 51] have reported that ethanol can inhibit the activity of the fatty acid desaturases, particularly Δ5 and Δ6 desaturase, which would be consistent with a decrease in long-chain polyunsaturates. Furthermore, ethanol exposure for a period of months [52] or for as short a duration as 3 h [53] can lead to reductions in tissue concentrations of both 22:6n3 and 20:4n6 under certain experimental conditions. It should be noted, however, that at least two studies [54, 55] have reported ethanol-induced increases in 22:6n3. It is possible that different experimental methodologies (i.e. species and strain studied, type of diet used, and pattern of severity of ethanol administration) account for some of these discrepancies. For example, one study reported that rats exhibited decreases in liver mitochondrial 22:6n3 following long-term ethanol consumption only when fed a high-fat diet (34% calories from fat as opposed to less than 5% in the low-fat group) [52]. In a recent study in which the fatty acid composition of the diet was manipulated, both 22:6n3 and 20:4n6 were decreased in rat synaptic membranes when the diet contained low levels of ω3 fatty acids but not if it contained adequate amounts of either short- or long-chain ω3s [56].

The apparent interference with the compositional integrity of the brain with respect to polyunsaturates caused by chronic alcohol exposure raises questions about their normal accretion mechanisms. This is a complex process involving many steps including absorption, elongation, desaturation, transport, complexation with lipoproteins, acylation, uptake into target organs and the remodeling of complex lipids. Dietary fatty acids or other factors including vitamin and mineral levels which modulate any of these processes may have an important influence. In addition, there are important species differences in the extent to which they depend upon dietary sources of long-chain essential fatty acids.

Essential Fatty Acid Metabolism

Recently, there have been technical developments in the use of stable isotope-labelled fatty acids combined with gas chromatography/mass spectrometry (GC/MS) techniques which have greatly expanded the opportunities for in vivo research. Pawlosky et al. [57] have demonstrated that negative ion, chemical ionization mode GC/MS has subpicogram detection capability for the pentafluorobenzyl derivatives of fatty acids with an increase in sensitivity of 3–4 orders of magnitude over positive ion methods previously used for methyl ester derivatives. Also contributing to the overall increase in method sensitivity is the complete resolution of the deuterated fatty acids from the endogenous ones on capillary columns due to the presence of five deuterium atoms; those with only four deuterium atoms per molecule produce inadequate separation. The use of the latter leads to low levels of detectability as the deuterium-labelled metabolite has (approximately) the same retention and mass as the endogenous compound species with four 13-C atoms. Even though only a very small percentage of the endogenous fatty acid molecules have four natural abundance 13-C atoms, this still creates a detection problem due to the fact that the endogenous compound is at a very much higher concentration than the deuterium-labeled metabolite to be measured. This approach has led to a rapid advance in our understanding of the regulatory features involved in fatty acid metabolism.

Pawlosky et al. [58] have presented preliminary results concerning 18:2n6 and 18:3n3 metabolism in mice, rats, cats and rhesus monkeys. It was clear that all of these species were able to produce both 20:4n6 and 22:6n3 under the appropriate conditions. Dietary studies in the cat and monkey indicated that the level of long-chain unsaturated fatty acids consumed is a critical variable as the highest levels of desaturated products were observed in the plasma when these were fed at a low level. In cats, deuterium-labeled 20:4n6 and 22:5n3 could be detected in plasma and liver; however, no labeled 22:6n3 could be detected in these tissues. Since the D5-22:6n3 was detected in the brains of these kittens, it appeared that the brain was performing at least the desaturase step. This led to the hypothesis that one functional metabolic pathway for 22:6n3 supply to the brain involves the desaturation/elongation of 18:3n3 in the liver to form 22:5n3 that is then exported via the circulation to the brain. The brain uptake of this intermediate then allows for 22:6n3 formation using brain enzymes that are apparently not found or not active in the peripheral tissues of cats. This hypothesis also explains what has been a rather perplexing fatty acyl composition with respect to ω3 fatty acids, i.e. the lack of 18:3n3 and 20:5n3 in the brain and the presence of a small amount of 22:5n3 and a large amount of 22:6n3. The cat seems to be an extreme case in this respect and the quantitative importance of this pathway depends upon the distribution and amount of essential fatty acids in the diet and the metabolic capacity of the liver of other species. For example, it would not be expected to be of much importance where there is a high level of 22:6n3 in the diet or in a species wherein the liver forms and exports adequate amounts of 22:6n3.

The above discussion is not meant to preclude the possibility of 18:3n3 being an important source of brain 22:6n3. In fact, our studies have indicated that 18:3n3 is taken up into the brain in young rodents [58]. The subsequent time courses of the levels of deuterium-labeled 18:3n3, 20:5n3, 22:5n3 and 22:6n3 in the brain indicate that there is a precursor/product relationship and it therefore appears that 18:3n3 can be metabolized in the brain all the way to 22:6n3. Scott and Bazan [59] are clearly incorrect in their assertion that radioactive 18:3n3 is not taken up into the brain. They have also indicated that all of the 22:6n3 supplied to the brain is derived from 22:6n3 produced in the liver.

The examples given above provide two exceptions to the hypothesis of Scott and Bazan [59] and indicate that it is naive to discuss the importance of various metabolic routes of brain 22:6n3 formation without reference to the amounts and types of dietary fatty acids. Only when the rates of these various pathways are measured in various species under differing dietary conditions (including ω3-deficient and 18:3n3 only or 22:6n3-adequate) can we begin to understand the metabolic mechanisms used to supply brain and retinal 22:6n3. It is crucial that we now determine the amounts of 22:6n3 needed in early development and to what extent and at what age the 18:3n3 precursor may substitute for it. Of course, we must also study the accumulation of, and requirements for, other essential fats such as 20:4n6, as well.

Biological Mechanisms Underlying 22:6n3 Function

We must now turn to the question of 'What is the molecular function of 22:6n3 in the nervous system that is essential?' Salem and Niebylski [60] have recently considered this issue. The extraordinary molecular specificity of the ω3 deficiency syndrome in the nervous system, i.e. the fact that reciprocal substitution of 22:5n6 for 22:6n3 [61] cannot prevent lack of organ system functional changes dictates that a hypothesis must predict this as a central feature. This type of specificity is normally ascribed by biochemists only to the molecular recognition capabilities of proteins. It seemed reasonable to assume that there was an enzymatic product produced from 22:6n3 that could not use 22:5n6 as a substrate and that this product had potent biological activity in the nervous system. Cyclo-oxygenases (CO) and lipoxygenases (LO) provided just such enzymes and both types of activity had been described in brain using 20:4n6 as substrate. Moreover, the products were prostaglandins and leukotrienes, agents known to have powerful modulatory functions in many organ systems. It seemed that the most likely hypothesis then would be one in which a CO or LO product of 22:6n3 was made in brain and subserved an essential function. We have carefully examined this hypothesis and rejected it [60, 62]. There is a very low level of 22:6n3 peroxidation in the rat brain and this production is not enzymatically mediated as stereochemical analysis reveals that it is a racemic mixture [63, 64]. The exceptions to this rule that have been thus far observed are brain microvessels which contain a 12-S-lipoxygenase [65] and the pineal gland which contains lipoxygenases that form 22:6n3 products [62]. These products may subserve important functions in these locations, however, it appears unlikely that they can mediate the changes in brain and retinal functions observed above. It must be stated that this does not imply that LO products of 22:6n3 do not have important functions in the circulation where they are made at much higher levels [66–68].

Several questions immediately arise and explanations are required to reconcile assertions in the literature that LO is present in brain parenchyma. Most of the LO activity ascribed to brain in these reports can be explained by the failure to properly perfuse the brain to remove platelets and other blood cells which contain LO. The efficacy of LO inhibitors may also be explained in this way. However, the activity observed in the perfused brain is still sensitive to LO inhibitors [62]. This may be accounted for by the fact that these inhibitors are free radical scavengers and have antioxidant activity; thus they are expected to inhibit nonenzymatic oxidation reactions as well. The lack of activity towards 22:6n3 is not a result of substrate specificity as the LO products of 20:4n6 are also non-enzymatically formed in the perfused rat brain. These studies have been performed in the rat and it is possible that there are other mammalian species which do have brain and retinal LO activity. However, the burden of proof will be upon those supporting this hypothesis to demonstrate such activity.

Of course, it is quite possible that there is a 22:6n3 enzymatic product that has a crucial biological function in the brain that is as yet unknown. It may be the product of an enzyme system that has not yet been discovered. Indeed, it is difficult to pose this conjecture in an empirical fashion. Although the use of radioactively labeled 22:6n3 may be expected to yield information about any potential metabolite, the reality is that the analytical methods used may not be capable of properly extracting, derivatizing, chromatographically separating or detecting the putative metabolite. It seems that part of the excitement in this field stems from its difficult nature; from the likelihood that an answer to the question will require some fundamental advance in our knowledge of polyunsaturate function and neurochemistry. Perhaps a discovery of the magnitude of that of prostaglandins and leukotrienes will be made when this puzzle is solved.

At this time, a more prudent approach to this problem involves the function of the 22:6n3-containing phospholipids in membranes. Although this concept would have seemed unlikely 10 years ago, and still may to many, we propose that the most favored hypothesis involves the membrane functions of the 22:6n3 phospholipid. In our laboratory, we have demonstrated that there are differences in physical properties between liposomal membranes composed of various polyunsaturates [60]. For example, there are differences in the rotational correlation times of DPH in PC membranes at 5 °C between species containing 4 or 5 double bonds vs. those with 6. A fruitful area for future research, if we are to understand the 'ω3 deficiency syndrome', will be to understand the functions of various polyunsaturated phospholipids in membranes, in particular, the protein-lipid interactions.

Conclusions and Dietary Recommendations

Finally, nutritional requirements for ω3 fatty acids must be considered. Since we are now making the decision every day about what to put in infant formulas, it would seem wise to use our best knowledge to design the lipid composition given to our infants as the sole source of food. Although our knowledge is incomplete, it would seem prudent to include the ω3 and ω6 polyunsaturates at levels similar to that of human milk. Since both premature and full term babies are undergoing rapid brain growth, this recommendation should apply to both. The formulation should be the same with respect to saturates, monoenes, dienes and ω3 and ω6 polyunsaturates as human milk. The 20:4n6, 20:5n3 and 22:6n3 would be in the same ratios as is found in human milk. Although it is recognized that the composition of human milk can vary depending upon the mother's diet, a conservative approach may be taken, i.e. using the levels of PUFAs found in the milk of western women. It would also be prudent for the rest of the population to eat a reasonable balance between ω3 and ω6 PUFA. The best reference point that we can offer is the ratio eaten by Paleolithic man in wild foods; the PUFA/saturate ratio was estimated to be about 1.4 [69]. The ω6 to ω3 ratio of 5:1 or less, e.g. 1:1 may be a starting point for research regarding the optimal balance between these competing fatty acids for the general population.

References

1 Salem N Jr, Kim H-Y, Yergey JA: Docosahexanoic acid: Membrane function and metabolism; in Simopoulos AP, Kifer RR, Martin R (eds): Health Effects of Polyunsaturated Fatty Acids in Seafoods. New York, Academic Press, 1986, pp 263–317.

2 Salem N Jr: Omega-3 fatty acids: Molecular and biochemical aspects; in Spiller G, Scala J (eds): New Protective Roles of Selected Nutrients in Human Nutrition. New York, Liss, 1989, pp 213–332.

3 Uauy R, Birch E, Birch D, et al: Visual and brain function measurements in studies of n–3 fatty acid requirements of infants. J Pediatr 1992;120:S168–S180.
4 Innis SM: Essential fatty acids in growth and development. Prog Lipid Res 1991;30: 39–103.
5 Bourre JM, Francois M, Youyou A, et al: The effects of dietary α-linolenic acid on the composition of nerve membranes, enzymatic activity, amplitude in electrophysiological parameters, resistance to poisons and performance of learning tasks in rats. J Nutr 1989;119:1880–1892.
6 Enslen M, Milon H, Malnoë A: Effect of low intake of n–3 fatty acids during development on brain phospholipid fatty acid composition and exploratory behavior in rats. Lipids 1991;26:203–208.
7 Lamptey MS, Walker BL: A possible essential role for dietary linolenic acid in the development of the young rat. J Nutr 1976;106:86–93.
8 Mills DE, Ward RP, Young C: Effects of prenatal and early postnatal fatty acid supplementation on behavior. Nutr Res 1988;8:273–286.
9 Reisbick S, Neuringer M, Hasnain R, et al: Polydipsia in rhesus monkeys deficient in omega–3 fatty acids. Physiol Behav 1990;47:315–323.
10 Reisbick S, Neuringer M, Connor WE: Postnatal deficiency of omega–3 fatty acids in monkeys: fluid intake and urine concentration. Physiol Behav 1992;51:473–479.
11 Wainwright PE, Huang YS, Bulman-Fleming B, et al: The role of n–3 essential fatty acids in brain and behavioral development: A cross-fostering study in the mouse. Lipids 1991;26:37–45.
12 Yamamoto N, Hashimoto A, Takemoto Y, et al: Effect of the dietary α-linolenate/linoleate balance on lipid compositions and learning ability of rats. II. Discrimination process, extinction process, and glycolipid compositions. J Lipid Res 1988;29: 1013–1021.
13 Yamamoto N, Okaniwa Y, Mori S, et al: Effects of a high-linoleate and a high-a-linolenate diet on the learning ability of aged rats: Evidence against an autoxidation-related lipid peroxide theory of aging. J Gerontol Biol Sci 1991;46:B17–22.
14 Wainwright PE: Do essential fatty acids play a role in behavioral development? Neurosci Biobehav Rev 1992;16:193–205.
15 Connor WE, Neuringer M, Reisbick S: Essentiality of omega–3 fatty acids: Evidence from the primate model and implications for human nutrition; in Simopoulos AP, Kifer RR, Martin RE, Barlow SM (eds): Health Effects of ω3 Polyunsaturated Fatty Acids in Seafoods. World Rev Nutr Diet, vol 66. Basel, Karger, 1991, pp 118–132.
16 Werkman SH, Peeples JM, Carlson SE, et al: Vitamin A status at expected delivery and growth and developmental scores of preterm infants during year one. FASEB J 1991;5:A1072.
17 Lucas A, Morley R, Cole TJ, et al: Breast milk and subsequent intelligence quotient in children born preterm. Lancet 1992;339:261–264.
18 Holman RT, Johnson SB, Hatch TF: A case of human linolenic acid deficiency involving neurological abnormalities. Am J Clin Nutr 1982;35:617–623.
19 O'Brien JS, Sampson EL: Kinky hair disease. II. Biochemical studies. J Neuropathol Exp Neurol 1966;25:523–530.
20 Kishimoto Y, Radin NS, Tourtellotte WW, et al: Gangliosides and glycerophospholipids in multiple sclerosis white matter. Arch Neurol 1967;16:44–54.

21 Svennerholm L, Hagberg B, Haltia M, et al: Polyunsaturated fatty acid lipidosis. II. Lipid biochemical studies. Acta Pediatr Scand 1975;64:489–496.
22 Pullarkat RK, Patel VK, Brockerhoff H: Leukocyte docosahexaenoic acid in juvenile form of ceroid-lipofuscinosis. Neuropädiatrie 1978;9:127–130.
23 Martinez M: Developmental profiles of polyunsaturated fatty acids in the brains of normal infants and patients with peroxisomal diseases: Severe deficiency of docosahexaenoic acid in Zellweger's and Pseudo-Zellweger's syndromes; in Simopoulos AP, Kifer RR, Martin RE, Barlow SM (eds): Health Effects of ω3 Polyunsaturated Fatty Acids in Seafoods. World Rev Nutr Diet, vol 66. Basel, Karger, 1991, pp 87–102.
24 Bernsohn J, Stephanides LM: Aetiology of multiple sclerosis. Nature 1967;215:821–823.
25 Anderson RE, Landis DJ, Dudley PA: Essential fatty acid deficiency and renewal of rod outer segments in the albino rats. Invest Ophthalmol 1976;15:232–236.
26 Benolken RM, Anderson RE, Wheeler TG: Membrane fatty acids associated with the electrical response in visual excitation. Science 1973;182:1253–1255.
27 Wheeler TG, Benolken RM, Anderson RE: Visual membranes: Specificity of fatty acid precursors for the electrical response to illumination. Science 1975;188:1312–1314.
28 Connor WE, Neuringer M, Barstad L, et al: Dietary deprivation of linolenic acid in rhesus monkeys: Effects on plasma and tissue fatty acid composition and on visual function. Trans Assoc Am Phys 1984;97:1–9.
29 Connor WE, Neuringer M: The effects of n–3 fatty acid deficiency and repletion upon the fatty acid composition and function of the brain and retina; in Karnovsky ML, Leaf A, Bolls LC (eds): Biological Membranes: Aberrations in Membrane Structure and Function. New York, Liss, 1988, pp 275–294.
30 Birch DG, Birch EE, Hoffman DR, et al: Retinal development in very-low-birth-weight infants fed diets differing in omega-3 fatty acids. Invest Ophthalmol Visual Sci 1992;33:2365–2376.
31 Birch EE, Birch DG, Hoffman DR, et al: Dietary essential fatty acid supply and visual acuity development. Invest Ophthalmol Vis Sci 1992;33:in press.
32 Anderson RE, Maude MB, Lewis RA, et al: Abnormal plasma levels of polyunsaturated fatty acid in autosomal dominant retinitis pigmentosa. Exp Eye Res 1987;44: 155–159.
33 Anderson RE, Maude MB, Alvarez RA, et al: Plasma lipid abnormalities in the miniature poodle with progressive rod-cone degeneration. Exp Eye Res 1991;52: 349–355.
34 Anderson RE, Maude MB, Nilsson SEG, et al: Plasma lipid abnormalities in the Abyssinian cat with a hereditary rod-cone degeneration. Exp Eye Res 1991;53:415–417.
35 Olsen SF, Joensen HD: High liveborn birth weight in the Faroes: A comparison between birth weights in the Faroes and in Denmark. J Epidemiol Commun Health 1985;39:27–32.
36 Olsen SF, Hansen HS, Sørensen TIA, et al: Intake of marine fat, rich in (n–3)-polyunsaturated fatty acids, may increase birthweight by prolonging ingestion. Lancet 1986;ii:367–369.
37 Guesnet Ph, Pascal G, Durand G: Dietary a-linolenic acid deficiency in the rat. I.

Effects on reproduction and postnatal growth. Reprod Nutr Develop 1986;26:969–985.

38 Pax JB, Keeney M, Sampugna J: Linolenic acid and trans fatty acids affect survival of mouse pups. FASEB J 1991;5:A1446.

39 Smith SS, Neuringer M, Ojeda SR: Essential fatty acid deficiency delays the onset of puberty in the female rat. Endocrinology 1989;125:1650–1659.

40 Fayard JM, Timouyasse L, Guesnet P, et al: Dietary α-linoleic acid deficiency and early uterine development in female rats. J Nutr 1992;122:1529–1535.

41 Allen BR, Maurice PDL, Goodfield MW, et al: The effects on psoriasis of dietary supplementation with eicosapentaenoic acid. Br J Dermatol 1985;113:777.

42 Ziboh VA, Cohen KA, Ellis CN, et al: Effects of dietary supplementation of fish oil on neutrophil and epidermal fatty acids. Arch Dermatol 1986;122:1277–1282.

43 Bjørneboe A, Søyland E, Bjørneboe G-EA, et al: Effect of fatty acid supplement to patients with atopic dermatitis. J Intern Med 1989;225:233–236.

44 Bjørneboe A, Smith AK, Bjørneboe G-EA, et al: Effect of dietary supplementation with n–3 fatty acids on clinical manifestations of psoriasis. Br J Dermatol 1988;118: 77–83.

45 Bjerve KS: α-linolenic acid deficiency in adult women. Nutr Rev 1987;45:15–19.

46 Watanabe T: Lipid nutrition in fish. Comp Biochem Physiol 1982;73B:3–15.

47 Satoh S, Poe WE, Wilson RP: Effect of dietary n–3 fatty acids on weight gain and liver fatty acid composition of fingerling channel catfish. J Nutr 1989;119:23–28.

48 Bjerve KS, Thoresen L, Fischer S: n–3 fatty acid deficiency in man: Effect of supplementing with ethyl linolenate and long-chain n–3 fatty acids; in Lands WEM (ed): Proceedings of the AOCS Short Course on Polyunsaturated Fatty Acids and Eicosanoids. Champaign, American Oil Chemists Society, 1987, pp 392–394.

49 Salem N: Alcohol, fatty acids, and diet. Alcohol Health Res World 1989;13:211–218.

50 Nervi AM, Peluffo RO, Brenner RR: Effect of ethanol administration on fatty acid desaturation. Lipids 1980;15:263–268.

51 Wang DL, Reitz RC: Ethanol ingestion and polyunsaturated fatty acids. Effects on the acyl-CoA desaturases. Alcohol Clin Exp Res 1983;7:220–226.

52 Thompson JA, Reitz RC: Effects of ethanol ingestion and dietary fat levels on mitochondrial lipids in male and female rats. Lipids 1978;13:540–550.

53 Littleton JM, John GR, Grieve SJ: Alterations in phospholipid composition in ethanol tolerance and dependence. Alcohol Clin Exp Res 1979;3:50–56.

54 Curstedt T: Biosynthesis of molecular species of hepatic glycerophosphatides during metabolism of (1,1-$^2H_2$) ethanol in rats. Biochim Biophys Acta 1982;713:589–601.

55 Sun GY, Sun AY: Effect of chronic ethanol administration on phospholipid acyl groups of synaptic plasma membrane fraction isolated from guinea pig brain. Res Commun Chem Pathol Pharmacol 1979;24:405–408.

56 Zérouga M, Beaugé F, Niel E, et al: Interactive effects of dietary (n–3) polyunsaturated fatty acids and chronic ethanol intoxication on synaptic membrane lipid composition and fluidity in rats. Biochim Biophys Acta 1991;1086:295–304.

57 Pawlosky RJ, Sprecher HW, Salem N Jr: A high sensitivity negative ion GC-MS method for detection of desaturated and chain elongated products of deuterated linoleic and linolenic acids. J Lipid Res 1992; in press.

58 Pawlosky RJ, Sprecher HW, Salem N Jr: Metabolism of essential fatty acids in mammals; in Sinclair A, Gibson R (eds): Proceedings of the Third International Conference on Essential Fatty Acids and Eicosanoids. Champlain, American Oil Chemists Society, 1992, in press.
59 Scott BL, Bazan NG: Membrane docosahexaenoate is supplied to the developing brain and retina by the liver. Proc Natl Acad Sci USA 1989;86:2903–2907.
60 Salem N Jr, Niebylski CD: An evaluation of alternative hypotheses involved in the biological function of docosahexaenoic acid in the nervous system; in Sinclair A, Gibson R (eds): Proceedings of the Third International Conference on Essential Fatty Acids and Eicosanoids. Champlain, American Oil Chemists Society, 1992, in press.
61 Galli C, Trzeciak HI, Paoletti R: Effects of dietary fatty acids on the fatty acid composition of brain ethanolamine phosphoglyceride: Reciprocal replacement of n–6 and n–3 polyunsaturated fatty acids. Biochim Biophys Acta 1971;248:449–454.
62 Kim H-Y, Sawazaki S, Salem N Jr: Lipoxygenation of polyunsaturated fatty acids in rat brain? in Sinclair A, Gibson R (eds): Proceedings of the Third International Conference on Essential Fatty Acids and Eicosanoids. Champlain, American Oil Chemists Society, 1992, in press.
63 Kim H-Y, Karanian JW, Shingu T, et al: Stereochemical analysis of hydroxylated docosahexaenoates produced by human platelet and rat brain homogenate. Prostaglandins 1990;40:473–490.
64 Kim H-Y, Sawazaki S, Salem N: Lipoxygenation in rat brain? Biochem Biophys Res Commun 1991;174:729–734.
65 Moore SA, Giordano MJ, Kim H-Y, et al: Brain microvessel 12-hydroxyeicosatetraenoic acid (12-HETE) is the (S) enantiomer and is lipoxygenase-derived. J Neurochem 1991;57:922–929.
66 Karanian JW, Kim H-Y, Shingu T, et al: Smooth muscle effects of hydroxylated docosahexaenoates produced from human platelet. Biomed Biochim Acta 1988;47: S79–82.
67 Karanian JW, Kim H-Y, Shingu T, et al: Cardiovascular properties of hydroxylated docosahexaenoates; in Schror K, Sinzinger M (eds): Prostaglandins in Clinical Research: Cardiovascular System. New York, Liss, 1989, pp 511–515.
68 Karanian JW, Kim H-Y, Salem N Jr: Physiological functions of hydroxydocosahexaenoic acid; in Sinclair A, Gibson R (eds): Proceedings of the Third International Conference on Essential Fatty Acids and Eicosanoids. Champlain, American Oil Chemists Society, 1992, in press.
69 Eaton SB, Konner M: Paleolithic nutrition. A consideration of its nature and current implications. N Engl J Med 1985;312:283–289.

Norman Salem, Jr., Chief, Laboratory of Membrane Biochemistry & Biophysics,
DICBR, NIAAA, ADAMHA, 10/3C103, 9000 Rockville Pike,
Bethesda, MD 20892 (USA)

Simopoulos AP (ed): Nutrition and Fitness in Health and Disease.
World Rev Nutr Diet. Basel, Karger, 1993, vol 72, pp 148–164

Dietary Fiber and Health

A. Stewart Truswell

Human Nutrition Unit, University of Sydney, Australia

Chemical, experimental and epidemiological evidence accumulates on the relations between dietary fiber intake and health or susceptibility to disease. Our concepts have evolved from the 1972 vision of Burkitt et al. [1] and Trowell's group [2, 3].

Fiber Is Difficult to Define

There are two main alternative definitions. One is biological. 'Dietary fibre' was first used by Hipsley [4] as a shorthand term for the constituents of plant cell walls (which he thought might be protective against toxaemia of pregnancy). Trowell [5] defined dietary fiber as 'the residue of plant foods that resist digestion by the alimentary enzymes of man ...' This adds to cell wall material (phloem and xylem) various indigestible storage polysaccharides. Some of these polysaccharides have been tested and used in extracted, purified form, which is almost the opposite of the concept of unrefined plant foods [6].

When we need to quantify nutrients and other substances in foods we use chemical analysis. Cummings [7] proposed a chemical definition of 'nonstarch polysaccharides plus lignin'. There is much more of the former. But there are other indigestible substances that we eat in plant cell walls, e.g. phytate, saponins, lectins, browning products, tannins, silica, protein, cutin, suberin, waxes, resistant starch, etc. [8]. The structure of plant material also has physiological effects in the gut [9].

Different Types of Fiber Have Different Physiological Effects

The original hypothesis implied that all dietary fiber had the same physiological and protective effects. Research has subsequently shown that types of fiber differ markedly in their effects in the small intestine on the rise of blood glucose after a meal [10], on plasma cholesterol [11], on transit time [12], on fermentability in the large intestine [7] and in relieving constipation [13].

Measurement of Fiber in Foods Is a Complex Operation and Not Yet Standardized

There are two major approaches with variations for each. One approach is chemical. After extracting lipids with ether, then free sugars with hot aqueous methanol, Southgate [14] digested the starch with takadiastase then separated dietary fiber by differential solubility in acid into cellulose and hemicelluloses, quantified by chemical methods for hexoses, pentoses and uronic acids (i.e. pectin). The residue, insoluble in 12 *M*, sulphuric acid was lignin. This procedure was modified by Englyst and Cummings [15], who introduced more reliable enzymes for digesting the starch, parallel flows to speed up the work and quantitation of the sugar residues by gas chromatography.

This method provides information about the different types of fiber but is a lot of work and may not reflect what happens in the gut. For food standards there is a need for a simpler, coarse tuning method. The enzymatic-gravimetric approach was introduced by Hellendoorn et al. [16] who defined dietary fiber as ‘the part of the food which is not solubilised after the most energetic enzymatic treatment’. Essentially, the residue after enzymatic digestion of starch and protein in the defatted food was weighed and, corrected for ash, this weight represents the total dietary fiber. The enzymatic approach has been improved by Prosky et al. [17, 18] and now distinguishes ‘soluble’ and ‘insoluble’ fiber. This method is simpler and cheaper and may (at least partly) reflect the digestive conditions in the upper gastrointestinal tract. The more complicated chemical fractionation can be used for research purposes. However, the Prosky et al. [18] method includes some resistant starch and gives higher values for dietary fiber in some foods than the Englyst method [19]. Either of these two approaches is going to be used in major analytical laboratories, with the Englyst (which can be further streamlined) preferred in the UK where it has been developed. Of other earlier methods the detergent/filtration method [20] is less suitable for human foods than for ruminants feeds [21] (for which it was originally developed) and 'crude fiber' is meaningless and obsolete.

Different methods have been used for present food tables and for nutrient labelling of foods. The Englyst and enzymatic-gravimetric methods have evolved through several modifications.

Insoluble Fiber, which Roughly Corresponds to Cellulose and Part of the Hemicelluloses, Increases Fecal Bulk and Helps to Relieve Constipation

Stool weight is increased by a number of types of fiber and fiber-rich foods [22]. Insoluble types of fiber such as wheat bran tend to produce the greatest increase on fecal weight and shorten mouth-to-anus transit time. Soluble fiber types such as pectin and gums have little or no effect on transit time and less effect on fecal weight. One mechanism for the increase in fecal weight is the water-holding property of fiber (such as wheat bran) that is not fermented in the colon. Another is fermentation of part of the polysaccharide, with increase of bacterial mass and associated water in the bowel. 'Soluble' types of fiber such as pectin and guar gum are largely fermented, so little of the original material passes on to the feces. Lignin is not fermented and cellulose is partly fermented. Hemicellulose, notably the arabinoxylan of wheat fiber, is more effective in increasing fecal bulk than cellulose [23]. Even with wheat fiber there are important effects of particle size and physical form. Coarse bran gives a greater stool weight than fine bran [24]. Wholemeal bread, unless it is very coarse, has no effect on stool weight [25].

Effects of Viscous/Soluble Fiber on the Upper Gastrointestinal Tract

Some types of fiber are viscous, not fibrous. Well studied examples are pectin, guar gum and the β-glucan of oat meal (or bran). In general viscous polysaccharides slow the emptying of fluids from the stomach [26]. This has been applied in treatment of the dumping syndrome [27]. Of more general application is the reduced glycemic response to carbohydrate meals when large doses of viscous fiber are taken, such as pectin or guar [28]. Various preparations of guar granules or food with guar incorporated have been used in some clinics as a second-line pharmaceutical treatment of diabetes [29, 30]. The main mechanism for the glucose-reducing effect of guar is thought to be viscous interference with movement of glucose in the jejunum [31]. The effect of guar on blood glucose is less consistent than the effect on plasma cholesterol [32].

A few years ago there were reports of improved control in diabetic patients on 'high carbohydrate, high fiber diets' [33, 34]. There is now much less emphasis on the fiber per se in therapeutic diets for diabetes since development of the concept of a glycemic index [35]. Fiber is only one of several variables that determine the glycemic index [36]. Those high fiber diets had low patient acceptibility. The glycemic index does not correlate well with the dietary fiber content of foods [37]. It is the glycemic index that determines postprandial glucose concentrations; fiber is effective only if it is in foods with a low glycemic index [38]. We have reported improved glucose control in NIDDM on palatable diets of lower glycemic index foods compared with higher glycemic index foods in a 3/3-month crossover trial; total fiber was the same in the two diets [39].

Effects of Fiber on Plasma Cholesterol

Trowell [2] expected that wheat fiber would lower plasma cholesterol. It does not, in nearly all the 34 reports in the literature [40].

Generous intakes of soluble or viscous fiber tend to lower plasma cholesterol [40]. This is seen with supplements of purified pectin or guar gum or with oatmeal or oat bran (which contains oat gum, a viscous β-glucan). The effect is on low density lipoprotein cholesterol; HDL cholesterol and triglycerides do not change. This property has been somewhat oversold. The effective amounts of pectin and guar have usually been 15 g/day (5 g thrice daily with meals) and some investigators have not found the fall of plasma cholesterol on oat bran or meal [41]. The average lowering of cholesterol by oat fiber is quite small; oat bran has not been well defined (unlike wheat bran) and the content of soluble fiber in oats varies more than twofold [42].

There are two hypotheses for the mechanism of action of viscous fiber. Interference with reabsorption of bile acids by viscous ileal contents is better supported by the evidence [40] than the alternative hypothesis of inhibition of hepatic cholesterol synthesis by volatile fatty acids produced by fermentation of fiber in the large bowel and absorbed into the inferior mesenteric vein.

With whole foods other than oats, modest but significant reductions of plasma cholesterol have been reported on large intakes of vegetable foods when fat intake was maintained the same between experimental and control diets [43–45]. The most likely active constituent of mixed vegetable foods, is pectin. With high intakes of vegetable foods, if the rest of the diet is not controlled, larger falls of plasma cholesterol have been seen. This is the *indirect* effect: high fiber foods are low in saturated fat and tend to displace it from the diet.

'Soluble' Dietary Fiber Is Only a Rough Measure of Viscous Fiber

Pectins, the β-glucan of oats and some other polysaccharides produce colloidal sols in aqueous solution. Solubility is often dependent on pH and ionic strength and can be dependent on specific cations such as calcium. Large differences in the distribution of dietary fiber between soluble and insoluble fractions can result from different methods or variations in the method [46, 47]. It is not generally recognized that pectins are extracted into the insoluble as well as the soluble fiber fraction.

Fiber May Increase Satiety and Protect against Gallstones and Diverticulitis

In short-term experiments, inclusion of fiber can be shown to increase *satiety* or delay the return of hunger after a meal [9, 49, 50]. This is not always seen and presumably depends on the type of fiber and conditions of the experiment. Long-term effects on body weight are more difficult to demonstrate. High fiber foods need more chewing and tend to be bulky. There is a small increase in fecal excretion of energy on high fiber diets [51]. Double-blind trials with fiber supplements have shown greater weight loss in the fiber-tablet group [52]. The bigger question is whether, as Burkitt and Trowell [53] thought people eating plenty of high fiber *foods* have some protection from obesity.

The possibility that low fiber intake is one cause of *gallstones* goes back to the rarity of gallstones in Africa where fiber intakes are high [53].

Case-control studies in homogenous populations have given little support to the hypothesis [54]. Experimentally, when wheat bran is added to the diet the cholesterol saturation index of bile is usually lowered [55]. This is because the proportion of deoxycholic acid falls [56] due to the fall of pH in the large intestine from fermentation of polysaccharides to volatile fatty acids which inhibits the conversion of cholic acid to deoxycholic acid. Less of this bile acid is therefore reabsorbed and secreted into the bile. This forms micelles which can hold more cholesterol solubilized. However, addition of bran to the diet of patients whose gallstones had been dissolved by medical treatment did not prevent recurrence [57].

Painter and Burkitt [58] first suggested that *diverticular disease* of the colon, apparently new in this century [59] and rare in Black Africans results from insufficient consumption of fiber. Diverticulosis is the first disease in which a high fiber intake was claimed to have a therapeutic effect [60]. In England, the disease is significantly less common in vegetarians [61]. Case-control studies in Japan and Greece have shown lower fiber intakes in the cases [62, 63] but these were symptomatic hospital patients. The only study of asymptomatic cases, found by population screening, showed lower fiber intakes only in the cases over 60 years of age [61]. In subsequent controlled therapeutic trials, bran was clearly better than placebo in surgical cases [64] but not in a trial in medical patients [65]. It has been suggested that symptomatic diverticular disease is a variant of irritable bowel syndrome in people who happen to have diverticulosis.

Fermentation of Dietary Fiber in the Colon

The colon contains about a trillion bacteria, weighing up to 200 g, of many and varied species, mostly anaerobic. They ferment most of the carbohydrate that comes into the cecum, whether it is digestible by human intestinal enzyme or not. Cummings [66] estimates that on a Western diet bacteria in the large bowel ferment 20–40 g of carbohydrate per day – non-starch polysaccharides, resistant starch and indigestible oligosaccharides (e.g. in legumes). In the process about 200–400 mmol of volatile (or short chain) fatty acids are produced, acetic, propionic and butyric. These lower the pH of the colonic contents and are mostly absorbed across the mucosa into the portal venous system. Hydrogen and methane gases are also produced and detectable in the breath. Lignin is not fermented. Cellulose is incompletely fermented, as is the arabinoxylan of wheat. Most other forms of fiber (e.g. pectin) are completely or almost completely fermented [67].

The consequences of this fermentation are still being worked out but some are already known. One is that the energy of the carbohydrate in dietary fiber is not 'unavailable'. The metabolizable energy of mixed dietary fiber is now estimated at around 2 kcal (8.4 kJ) per gram [68], about half that for available carbohydrate because some of the energy goes into synthesis of bacteria, lost in the feces. Another consequence of the fermentation is that butyrate is available for utilization by colonic epithelial cells, which metabolize this substrate in preference to glucose [69]. The short chain fatty acids stimulate absorption of salt and water. Fermentation changes the pattern of rearbsorbed bile acids; less deoxycholic is formed and absorbed. The short-chain fatty acids may have metabolic effects after absorption or influence liver metabolism. One possibility is a small increase of plasma cholesterol, attributable to acetate absorption [70].

Reduced Risk of Large Bowel Cancer?

This is the biggest possible benefit of dietary fiber. By increasing the bulk of colonic contents and speeding transit time dietary fiber should cause dilution of potential carcinogens in the colon and reduce the time they are in contact with the epithelium [71]. Other theoretical advantages are reduced bacterial production of mutagens at the lower pH in the colon and increased production of butyrate which may lessen the risk of malignant change [72]. The increased hydrogen production should act as a reducing agent and reduce free radical damage [73].

Animal experiments have given confusing results [74] but here the carcinoma is induced by feeding a potent carcinogen such as dimethylhydrazine, very different from the pathogenesis in man. The published human observational epidemiological studies up to 1988 have been critically reviewed by Trock et al. [75]. Among these were 23 case-control studies, of which 9 provide strong support for a protective effect of fiber and 6 provide moderate support; 6 had equivocal results that neither support or refute a protective effect and 2 strongly support a lack of protective effect of fiber. In addition, there are two large prospective studies. Hirayama's study on 265,000 Japanese provided strong support for a protective effect of fiber, and the study by Willett et al. [77] on over 88,000 US nurses gives at the first report only some suggestion that a high intake of fiber-containing fruits may contribute to a lower risk of colon cancer. Trock et al. [75] were able to perform meta-analysis on 16 of the case-control studies that provided enough data. These indicate a probable protective effect of total fiber *and* of vegetables. It may not necessarily, or only, be the fiber that is protective in vegetables.

These results are not conclusive but case-control studies like this have many limitations. Data for fiber content of foods is incomplete today and was worse when some of these studies were done; some even used 'crude fiber' values. There are a number of possible confounders, such as a correlation between energy and fiber intakes. Some studies considered colon cancer alone, others considered rectal as well as colonic cancers (the effect of beer appears to be different between these two sites). Positive associations between fat and meat intake and colon cancer have been demonstrated more clearly [77], but these are easier to define in foods. Recently, the possibility has been recognized that resistant starch is also fermented in the colon [78] but was not estimated till now in the epidemiological studies. It forms more butyrate than most types of fiber.

Dietary Fiber and Estrogens

I don't think sex was among the many parts of the dietary fiber hypothesis in the early 1970s but it seems possible that relatively high intakes of some types of dietary fiber may lead to lower serum estrogens. Vegetarians have been found to have lower plasma estradiol and estrone than omnivores, both before and after the menopause and to excrete less estrone in the urine but more estrogens in feces [79–81]. The vegetarians were consuming less total fat and more dietary fiber. Fecal β-glucuronidase activity was significantly lower in the vegetarians; fecal estrogen excretion correlated well with (wet) weight of feces [80]. Much the same findings were obtained in a comparison of Caucasian Boston women and recent immigrants from SE Asia [82]. Serum estradiol was positively correlated with (total) fat intake ($r = 0.65$) and equally, negatively, correlated with dietary fiber intake ($r = -0.66$). Experimentally, US women who changed to a Pritikin diet, which is very low in fat and high in fiber showed a prompt reduction of plasma estradiol [83]. Low fat diets tend to be low in calories and high in fiber. Ingram et al. [84] report a modest fall of plasma estrogens on changing from a 40% to a prescribed 20% fat diet in premenopausal but not postmenopausal women. Estimated dietary fiber intakes were only 2 g/day higher on the low fat diet. Rose et al. [85] reported very similar changes on low fat diets with fiber maintained. Rose has subsequently mentioned that unpublished studies in his laboratory have shown that increased consumption of selected cereal brans, without changing fat intake, reduces fecal β-glucuronidase activity in pre-menopausal women [86], and a wheat bran supplement led to decreased plasma estrogen levels [87]. More controlled experiments with fiber (and fat intake unchanged) are clearly needed. Meanwhile, Adlercreutz et al. [88] report relatively high excretion of phyto-(anti-)estrogen, isoflavonoids in rural Japanese women who are known as a group to have low rates of breast cancer. This is another way in which plant foods can influence estrogen metabolism.

Some Effects of Dietary Fiber May Be Due to Associated Substances in Vegetable Foods

There are stimulants of intestinal motor activity in some foods, e.g. prunes contain derivatives of hydroxyphenylisatin [89]. Lowering of post-prandial glucose is achieved by slowly digested starch or sugar (fructose) as well as by viscous dietary fiber. Any protection from large intestinal cancer may come from anti-cancer substances in brassicas as well as dilution and fermentation in the colon. Antioxidants in plant foods, vitamins C and E and carotenoids may contribute to delaying atherosclerosis. Ulbricht and Southgate [90] think that the evidence for a protective effect of fiber is weaker than that now accumulating in favor of antioxidants.

Purified Concentrated Forms of Fiber versus Whole Foods

There are two possible nutrition strategies. One is to re-state in 1990 terms the original vision that we should not refine or dilute our plant foods. For Heaton [91] ‘dietary fibre is essentially the cell-wall material of plants. In the plant it fulfils a mechanical or structural role, providing its stiffening or skeleton. It is in fact the very architecture of the plant ...’ For Eastwood and Morris [92] ‘the physiological effects of dietary fiber depend predominantly on physical properties that do not relate in any simple way to chemical composition'. The relevance of physical shape, as opposed to chemistry is illustrated by the laxative properties of indigestible plastic particles [93].

Some of the histological structure of bran can still be seen in feces [94].

On the other hand, purified preparations have been more suitable for research on the effects of fiber. They can separate the effects of a particular type of fiber from other types of fiber and other components in plant foods. They even lend themselves to double-blind trials. Food manufacturers may then enrich their products with a bit more fiber, sometimes from the same or similar food, sometimes not, and pharmaceutical companies have a variety of fiber preparations in the pharmacopoeia. Some of the latter are undoubtedly effective in a limited role but this is industrializing the original concept of dietary fiber which was urging us to return to less processed foods.

Fecal Losses of Divalent Cations

The most important of the possible adverse effects of increased intake of dietary fiber is increased fecal excretion of iron, calcium, zinc and magnesium, all very critical inorganic nutrients. Rossander et al. [95] have reviewed the research on this problem and conclude that it is the associated phytate which reduces iron and zinc absorption, not fiber per se. Vegetables and fruit contain varying amounts of ascorbic acid (and other organic acids) which enhance iron absorption. Pharmaceutical preparations of dephytinized wheat bran are available in Sweden.

Recommendations by National Nutrition Committees

National nutrition committees are recommending adult intakes of 25–30 g/day total dietary fiber or 3 g fiber per MJ, e.g. in the Netherlands [96], the Nordic Countries [97], New Zealand [98], Germany [99] and in the report for WHO Europe [100]. In the UK and in the report for WHO, Geneva, a quantitative recommendation is expressed in different numbers, 16–24 g per day as non-starch polysaccharides [101, 102]. 'The 16 and 24 g levels of non-starch polysaccharides are consistent with estimates of about 27 and 40 g of total fiber, which included other fiber components' [102]. All these numbers imply significant increases in fiber in developed countries. In other countries expert committees recommend instead an increase of (or 'eat plenty of') cereals (preferably wholegrain), vegetables (including legumes) and fruits. These guidelines, which do not set a numerical target for fiber are current in the USA [103–106], Australia [107] and Singapore [108].

Lastly

For some subgroups of people, an increased fiber intake may not be helpful. These include long-distance athletes and infants.

References

1 Burkitt DP, Walker AR, Painter NS: Effect of dietary fibre on stools and transit times and its role in the causation of disease. Lancet 1972;ii:1408–1412.
2 Trowell HC: Ischaemic heart disease and dietary fiber. Am J Clin Nutr 1972;25: 926–932.
3 Burkitt DP, Trowell HC (eds): Refined Carbohydrate Foods and Disease. London, Academic Press, 1975.
4 Hipsley EH: 'Dietary fibre' and pregnancy toxaemia. Br Med J 1953;ii:420–422.
5 Trowell HC: The development of the concept of dietary fiber in human nutrition. Am J Clin Nutr 1978;31:S3–S11.
6 Heaton KW: Dietary fibre: Concepts and definitions; in Wallace G, Bell L (eds): Fibre in Human and Animal Nutrition, bull 20. Wellington, Royal Society of New Zealand, 1983, pp 19–21.
7 Cummings JH: Dietary fibre. Br Med Bull 1981;37:65–70.
8 Kay RM: Dietary fiber. J Lipid Res 1982;23:221–242.
9 Haber GB, Heaton KW, Murphy D, Burroughs L: Depletion and disruption of dietary fibre. Effects on satiety, plasma-glucose and serum insulin. Lancet 1977;ii: 679–682.
10 Wolever TMS, Jenkins DJA: Effect of dietary fiber and foods on carbohydrate metabolism; in Spiller GA (ed): CRC Handbook on Dietary Fiber in Human Nutrition. Boca Raton, CRC Press, 1986, pp 87–119.
11 Truswell AS, Kay RM: Absence of effect of bran on blood lipids. Lancet 1975;i: 922–923.
12 Cummings JH, Southgate DAT, Branch W, Houston H, Jenkins DJA, James WPT: The colonic response to dietary fibre from carrot, cabbage, apple, bran and guar gum. Lancet 1978;i:5–9.
13 Heaton KW: Dietary fibre (Regular review). Br Med J 1990;300:1479–1480.

14 Southgate DAT: Determination of carbohydrates in foods. II. Unavailable carbohydrates. J Sci Food Agric 1969;20:331–335.

15 Englyst HN, Cummings JH: Improved method for measurement of dietary fiber as non-starch polysaccharides in plant foods. J Assoc Off Anal Chem 1988;71:808–814.

16 Hellendoorn EW, Noordhoff MG, Slegman J: Enzymatic determination of the indigestible residue (dietary fibre) content of human food. J Sci Food Agric 1975;26: 1461–1468.

17 Prosky L, Asp N-G, Furda I, De Vries JW, Schweizer T, Harland B: Determination of total dietary fiber in foods, food products and total diets: Interlaboratory study. J Assoc Off Anal Chem, 1984;67:1044–1052.

18 Prosky L, Asp N-G, Schweizer TF, De Vries JW, Furda I: Determination of insoluble and total dietary fiber in foods and food products: Interlaboratory study. J Assoc Off Anal Chem 1988;71:1017–1023.

19 Englyst H, Cummings J: Dietary fibre and starch: Definition, classification and measurement; in Leeds AR, Burley VJ (eds): Dietary Fibre Perspectives – Reviews and Bibliography, 2. London, Libbey, 1990, pp 3–26.

20 Van Soest PJ, Wine RH: Use of detergents in the analysis of fibrous feeds. IV. Determination of plant cell-wall constituents. J Assoc Off Anal Chem 1967;50:50–55.

21 Asp N-G, Schweizer TF, Southgate DAT, Theander O: Dietary fibre analysis; in Kritchevsky D (ed): Dietary Fibre – A Component of Food: Nutritional Function in Health and Disease. Berlin, Springer, 1992, pp 57–101.

22 Cummings JH: The effect of dietary fiber on fecal weight and composition; in Spiller GA (ed): CRC Handbook of Dietary Fiber in Human Nutrition. Boca Raton, CRC Press, 1986, pp 211–280.

23 Williams RD, Olmsted WH: The effect of cellulose, hemicellulose and lignin on the weight of the stool. A contribution to the study of laxation in man. J Nutr 1936;11: 433–449.

24 Brodribb AJM, Groves C: Effect of bran particle size on stool weight. Gut 1978;19: 60–63.

25 Muller-Lissner SA: Effect of wheat bran on weight of stool and gastrointestinal transit time: A meta analysis. Br Med J 1988;296:615–617.

26 Holt S, Heading RC, Carter DC, Prescott LF, Tothill P: Effect of gel-forming fibre on gastric emptying and absorption of glucose and paracetamol. Lancet 1979;i:636–639.

27 Leeds AR, Ralphs DNL, Ebeid F, Metz G, Dilawari JB: Pectin in the dumping syndrome: Reduction of symptoms and plasma volume changes. Lancet 1981;i: 1075–1078.

28 Jenkins DJA, Goff DV, Leeds AR, Alberti KGMM, Wolever TMS, Gassull MA, Hockaday TDR: Unabsorbable carbohydrates and diabetes: Decreased post-prandial hyperglycaemia. Lancet 1976;ii:172–174.

29 Peterson DB, Mann JI: Guar: Pharmacological fibre or food fibre? Diabetic Med 1985;2:345–347.

30 Vinik AI, Jenkins DJA: Dietary fiber in management of diabetes. Diabetes Care 1988;11:160–173.

31 Uusutupa M, Siituone O, Savolainen K, Silvasti M, Penttila M, Parvioinen M: Metabolic and nutritional effects of long term use of guar gum in the treatment of non-insulin-dependent diabetes of poor metabolic control. Am J Clin Nutr 1989;49: 345–351.

32 Edwards CA, Blackman NA, Craigen L, et al: Viscosity of food gums determined in vitro related to their hypoglycemic actions. Am J Clin Nutr 1987;46:72–77.

33 Anderson JW, Ward K: High-carbohydrate, high-fiber diets for insulin-treated men with diabetes mellitus. Am J Clin Nutr 1979;32:2312–2321.

34 Simpson HCR, Simpson RW, Lousley S, et al: A high carbohydrate leguminous fibre diet improves all aspects of diabetic control. Lancet 1981;i:1–5.

35 Jenkins DJA, Wolever TMS, Taylor RH, et al: Glycemic index of foods: A physiological basis for carbohydrate exchange. Am J Clin Nutr 1985;42:1192–1196.

36 Thorburn AW, Brand JC, Truswell AS: The glycaemic index of foods. Med J Austr 1986;144:580–582.

37 Jenkins DJA, Wolever TMS, Jenkins AL, Lee R, Wong GS, Josse R: Glycemic response to wheat products: Reduced response to pasta but no effect of fiber. Diabetes Care 1983;6:155–159.

38 Tattersall RB, Mansell P: Fibre in the management of diabetes: Benefits of fibre itself are uncertain. Br Med J 1990;300:1336.

39 Brand JC, Colagiuri S, Crossman S, Allen A, Roberts DCK, Truswell AS: Low glycemic index foods improve long-term glycemic control in NIDDM. Diabetes Care 1991;14:95–101.

40 Truswell AS, Beynen AC: Dietary fibre and plasma lipids: potential for prevention and treatment of hyperlipidaemias; in Kritchevsky D (ed): Dietary Fibre – A Component of Food: Nutritional Function in Health and Disease. Berlin, Springer, 1992, pp 295–332.

41 Leadbetter J, Ball MJ, Mann JI: Effect of increasing quantities of oat bran in hypercholesterolemic people. Am J Clin Nutr 1991;54:841–845.

42 Asp N-G, Mattson B, Önning G: Variation in dietary fibre, β-glucan, protein, fat and hull content of oats grown in Sweden 1987–1989. Eur J Clin Nutr 1992;46:31–37.

43 Keys A, Anderson JT, Grande F: Diet-type (fats constant) and blood lipids in man. J Nutr 1968;70:257–266.

44 Stasse-Wolthuis M, Albers HFF, van Jeveren JGC, de Jong JW, Hautvast JGAJ, Hermus RJJ, Katan MB, Brydon WG, Eastwood MA: Influence of dietary fiber from vegetables and fruits, bran or citrus pectin on serum lipids, fecal lipids and colonic function. Am J Clin Nutr 1980;33:1745–1756.

45 Lewis B, Katan M, Merkx I, Miller NE, Hammett K, Kay RM, Nobels A, Swan AV: Towards an improved lipid-lowering diet; additive effects of changes in nutrient intake. Lancet 1981;ii:1310–1313.

46 Marlett JA, Chester JG, Longacre MJ, Bogdanske JJ: Recovery of soluble dietary fiber is dependent on the method of analysis. Am J Clin Nutr 1989;50:479–485.

47 Monro JA: Dietary fiber pectic substances: source of discrepancy between methods of fiber analysis. J Food Composition Anal 1991;4:88–99.

48 Marlett JA: Dietary fiber: Definition and determination. Proceedings of the 14th International Congress of Nutrition (Seoul, Korea, Aug 20–25, 1989), Keynote, Plenary and Symposium Lectures, pp 194–197.

49 Brand JC, Holt S, Saveny C, Hansky J: Plasma glucose correlates inversely with satiety and CCK. Proc Nutr Soc Aust 1990;15:209.
50 Burley VJ, Leeds AR, Blundell JE: The effect of high and low-fibre breakfasts on hunger, satiety and food intake in a subsequent meal. Int J Obes 1987;11:(suppl 1): 87–93.
51 Southgate DAT, Durnin JVGA: Calorie conversion factors: an experimental reassessment of the factors used in the calculation of the energy value of human diets. Br J Nutr 1970;24:517–535.
52 Ryttig KR, Leeds AR, Rössner S: Dietary fibre in the management of overweight – an update; in Leeds AR, Burley VJ (eds): Dietary Fibre Perspectives – Reviews and Bibliography, 2. London, Libbey, 1990, pp 87–99.
53 Burkitt DP, Trowell HC (eds): Refined Carbohydrate Foods and Disease. Some Implications of Dietary Fibre. London, Academic Press, 1975.
54 Pixley F, Mann JI: Dietary factors in the aetiology of gallstones: A case control study. Gut 1988;29:1511–1515.
55 Heaton KW: Effect of dietary fibre on biliary lipids; in Barbara L, Bianchi Porro G, Cheli R, Lipkin M (eds): Nutrition in Gastrointestinal Disease. New York, Raven Press, 1987, pp 213–222.
56 Marcus SN, Heaton KW: Deoxycholic acid and the pathogenesis of gallstones. Gut 1988;29:522–533.
57 Hood K, Gleeson D, Ruppin D, Dowling H: Can gallstone recurrence be prevented? The British/Belgian post-dissolution trial. Gastroenterology 1988;94:A548.
58 Painter NS, Burkitt DP: Diverticular disease of the colon. A deficiency disease of Western civilization. Br Med J 1971;ii:450–454.
59 Cleave TL, Campbell GD, Painter NS: Diabetes, Coronary Thrombosis and the Saccharine Disease, ed 2. Bristol, John Wright, 1969.
60 Painter NS, Almeida AZ, Colebourne KW: Unprocessed bran in treatment of diverticular disease of the colon. Br Med J 1972;ii:137–140.
61 Gear JSS, Ware A, Fursdon P, Mann JI, Nolan DH, Brodribb AJM, Vessey MP: Symptomless diverticular disease and intake of dietary fibre. Lancet 1979;i:511–514.
62 Ohta M, Ishiguro S, Iwane S, Nakaji S, Sano M, Tsuchida S, Aisawa T, Yoshida Y: An epidemiological study on the relationship between intake of dietary fibre and colonic diseases. Jpn J Gastroenterol 1985;82:51–57.
63 Manousos P, Day NE, Tzonou A, Papadimitriou C, Kapetanakis A, Polychronopoulou-Trichopulou A, Trichopoulos D: Diet and other factors in the aetiology of diverticulosis: an epidemiological study in Greece. Gut 1985;26:544–549.
64 Brodribb AJM: Treatment of symptomatic diverticular disease with a high-fibre diet. Lancet 1977;i:664–666.
65 Ornstein MH, Littlewood ER, Baird IM, Fowler J, North WRS, Cox AG: Are fibre supplements really necessary in diverticular disease of the colon? A controlled clinical trial. Br Med J 1981;282:1353–1356.
66 Cummings JH: Fermentation in the human large intestine: Evidence and implications for health. Lancet 1983;i:1206–1209.
67 Topping DL, Illman RJ: Bacterial fermentation in the human large bowel. Time to change from the roughage model of dietary fibre. Med J Aust 1986;144:307–309.

68 Livesey G: The energy value of carbohydrate and 'fibre' for man. Proc Nutr Soc Aust 1991;16:79–88.
69 Roediger WEW: Utilization of nutrients by isolated epithelial cells of the rat colon. Gastroenterology 1982;83:424–429.
70 Jenkins DJA, Wolever TMS, Jenkins A, et al: Specific types of colonic fermentation may raise low-density-lipoprotein-cholesterol concentrations. Am J Clin Nutr 1991; 54:141–147.
71 Burkitt D: Don't Forget Fibre in Your Diet. London, Martin Dunitz, 1979.
72 Sakata T, Yajima T: Influence of short chain fatty acids on the epithelial cell division of digestive tract. Q J Exp Physiol 1984;69:639–648.
73 Neale RJ: Dietary fibre and health: The role of hydrogen production. Med Hypotheses 1988;27:85–87.
74 The Report of the British Nutrition Foundation's Task Force: Complex Carbohydrates in Foods. London, Chapman & Hall, 1990.
75 Trock B, Lanza E, Greenwald P: Dietary fiber, vegetables and colon cancer: Critical review and meta-analysis of the epidemiologic evidence. J Natl Cancer Inst 1990;82: 650–661.
76 Hirayama T: A large scale cohort study of the relationship between diet and selected cancers of digestive organs; in Bruce WR, Correa P, Lipkin M,et al (eds): Gastrointestinal Cancer: Endogenous Factors. Cold Spring Harbour, Coldspring Harbour Laboratory, 1981, pp 409–429.
77 Willett WC, Stampfer MJ, Colditz GA, Rosner BA, Speizer FE: Relation of meat, fat and fiber intake to the risk of colon cancer in a prospective study among women. N Engl J Med 1990;323:1664–1672.
78 Cummings JH, Bingham SA: Dietary fibre and large bowel cancer. Proceedings of the 14th International Congress of Nutrition (Seoul, Korea Aug 20–25, 1989), Keynote, Plenary and Symposium Lectures, pp 202–205.
79 Goldin BR, Adlercreutz H, Dwyer JT, Swenson L, Warram JH, Gorbach SL: Effect of diet and excretion of estrogens in pre- and postmenopausal women. Cancer Res 1981;41:3771–3773.
80 Goldin BR, Adlercreutz H, Gorbach SL, Warram JH, Dwyer JT, Swenson L, Woods MN: Estrogen excretion patterns and plasma levels in vegetarian and omnivorous women. N Engl J Med 1982;307:1542–1547.
81 Shultz TD, Leklem JE: Nutrient intake and hormonal status of premenopausal vegetarian Seventh-day Adventists and premenopausal nonvegetarians. Nutr Cancer 1983:4:247–259.
82 Goldin BR, Adlercreutz H, Gorbach SL, Woods MN, Dwyer JT, Conlon T, Bohn E, Gershoff SN: The relationship between estrogen levels and diets of Caucasian American and Oriental immigrant women. Am J Clin Nutr 1986;44:945–953.
83 Heber D, Ashley JM, Leaf DA, Barnard RJ: Reduction of serum estradiol in postmenopausal women given free access to low-fat high-carbohydrate diet. Nutrition 1991;7:137–139.
84 Ingram DM, Bennett FC, Willcox D, de Klerk N: Effect of low-fat diet on female sex hormone levels. J Natl Cancer Inst 1987;79:1225–1229.
85 Rose DP, Boyar AP, Cohen C, Strong LE: Effect of a low-fat diet on hormone levels in women with cystic breast disease. I. Serum steroids and gonadotropins. J Natl Cancer Inst 1987;78:623–626.

86 Rose DP: Dietary fibre and breast cancer. Nutr Cancer 1990;13:1–8.
87 Rose DP: Breast cancer – role of fibre. Proceedings of Kellogg Nutrition Symposium (Sydney, Australia, May 2, 1990). Pagewood, NSW Kellogg (Australia) Pty Ltd, 1991.
88 Adlercreutz H, Honjo H, Higashi A, Fotsis T, Hämäläinen E, Hasegawa T, Okada H: Urinary excretion of lignans and isoflavonoid phytoestrogens in Japanese men and women consuming a traditional Japanese diet. Am J Clin Nutr 1991;54:1093–1100.
89 Passmore R, Eastwood MA: Davidson and Passmore Human Nutrition and Dietetics. Edinburgh, Churchill-Livingstone, 1986.
90 Ulbricht TLV, Southgate DAT: Coronary heart disease: Seven dietary factors. Lancet 1991;338:985–992.
91 Heaton KW: Review article. Dietary fibre in perspective. Hum Nutr 1983;37C: 151–170.
92 Eastwood MA, Morris MA: Physical properties that influence physiological function: A model for polymers along the gastrointestinal tract. Am J Clin Nutr 1992;55: 436–447.
93 Tomlin J, Read NW: Laxative properties of indigestible plastic particles. Br Med J 1988;297:1175–1176.
94 Schel JHN, Stasse-Wolthuis M, Katan MB, Willemse MTM: Structural changes in wheat bran after human digestion. Wageningen, Medelingen Landbouwhogeschool, 1980;80–14:1–9.
95 Rossander L, Sandberg A-S, Sandstrom B: The influence of dietary fibre on mineral absorption and utilization; in Kritchevsky D, Schweizer T (eds): Dietary Fibre – A Component of Food: Nutritional Function in Health and Disease. Berlin, Springer, 1992, pp 197–216.
96 Guidelines for a Healthy Diet (English version). Den Haag, Netherlands Nutrition Council, 1986.
97 Nordisk Ministerrad, Standing Nordic Committee on Food: Nordic Nutrition Recommendations, ed 2 (English version). Uppsala, National Food Administration, 1989.
98 Report of the Nutrition Taskforce: Food for Health. Wellington, Department of Health, 1991.
99 Deutsche Gesellschaft für Ernährung: Empfehlungen für die Nährstoffzufuhr 5. Überarbeitung. Umschau, Frankfurt/Main, 1991.
100 James WPT, Ferro-Luzzi A, Isaksson B, et al: Healthy nutrition: Preventing Nutrition Related Diseases in Europe. Copenhagen, WHO Regional Office for Europe, 1988.
101 Department of Health: Report of the Panel on Dietary Reference Values of the Committee on Medical Aspects of Food Policy. Dietary Reference Values for Food Energy and Nutrients for the United Kingdom. Report on Health and Social Subjects 41. London, HM Stationery Office, 1991.
102 Report of a WHO Study Group: Diet, Nutrition and the Prevention of Chronic Diseases. Technical Report Series 797. Geneva, World Health Organization, 1990.
103 The Surgeon General's Report on Nutrition and Health: DHHS (PHS) Publication 88-50210. Washington, US Department of Health & Human Services, 1988.

104 US Department of Agriculture and US Department of Health & Human Services: Nutrition and your Health: Dietary Guidelines for Americans, ed 3. Home & Garden Bulletin No. 232. Hyattsville, Human Nutrition Information Service, US Department of Agriculture, 1990.
105 Committee on Diet and Health, Food and Nutrition Board, National Research Council: Diet and Health. Implications for Reducing Chronic Disease Risk. Washington, National Academy Press, 1989.
106 Healthy People 2000: National Health Promotion and Disease Prevention Objectives. DHHS Publication No. PHS 91-50212. Washington, US Government Printing Office, 1991.
107 Report of the Panel to Review the Dietary Guidelines: Dietary Guidelines for Australians. Canberra, National Health and Medical Research Council, 1992.
108 Guidelines for a Healthy Diet: Recommendations of the National Advisory Committee on Foods and Nutrition. Singapore, Training & Health Education Department, Ministry of Health, 1989.

A. Stewart Truswell, MD, FRCP, Human Nutrition Unit, University of Sydney, Sydney, NSW 2006 (Australia)

Simopoulos AP (ed): Nutrition and Fitness in Health and Disease.
World Rev Nutr Diet. Basel, Karger, 1993, vol 72, pp 165–176

Vitamin E and Exercise: Aspects of Biokinetics and Bioavailability

Andreas M. Papas

Eastman Chemical Company, Kingsport, Tenn., USA

Introduction

Physical activity, and especially strenuous exercise, accelerates production of free radicals and may induce immune reactions identical to the acute-phase response to infection and injury [1–5]. As a major biological antioxidant, vitamin E is an essential component of the body's defense against the harmful effects of free radicals [6] and recent studies suggest that it protects muscles and other tissues against oxidative injury [1–5, 7, 8]. Thus, as discussed by Dr. Simon-Schnass in her paper in volume 71, vitamin E plays an important role in exercise and physical fitness.

Biopotencies for various vitamin E forms, established primarily by the 'fetal resorption-gestation' method in rats [9] have been assumed to predict bioavailability in humans and other species. Recent research, however, documented major species differences in the utilization of various forms [10, 11]. Within the same species, uptake and elimination by various tissues differ dramatically [6]. Thus, its potential is affected by absorption, transport, tissue uptake and elimination.

This paper discusses aspects of bioavailability and biokinetics of vitamin E in humans which are important in understanding its role in exercise and fitness.

Background Information

Compounds with Vitamin E Activity

Vitamin E has become synonymous with α-tocopherol, because this form exhibits the highest potency and is the predominant form in human and animal tissues [12, 13]. In addition to α-, three other naturally occurring tocopherols, designated as β-, γ- and δ-tocopherol, possess some vitamin E activity. Tocopherols consist of a chroman ring and a long saturated phytyl chain; they differ only in the number and position of the methyl group on the chroman ring. A related family of four compounds, designated as α-, β-, γ-, and δ-tocotrienols are also found in nature and differ from the corresponding tocopherols only in the side chain (saturated in tocopherols, unsaturated in tocotrienols). Only α-tocotrienol possesses measurable vitamin E activity. The chemical structures of tocopherols and tocotrienols are shown in figure 1a, b.

Total tocopherol content of foods and the relative proportion of each vary widely [14]. Good sources include vegetable oils, wheat germ, nuts and green leafy vegetables. In contrast, meat, fish, animal fats and most fruits and vegetables contain little vitamin E.

Chiral Forms

Tocopherols have three asymmetric carbons at the 2, 4′ and 8′ positions. In nature, biosynthesis of tocopherols yields only the RRR-stereoisomer. In contrast, tocopherols produced by chemical synthesis, by condensing isophytol with tri-, di- or monomethylhydroquinone are racemic (all-rac) mixtures of 8 stereoisomers. While all four tocopherols can be produced by chemical synthesis, only all-rac-α-tocopherol has commercial significance (fig. 1c). All four tocopherols are used as food antioxidants and/or for their vitamin E activity.

The nomenclature of tocopherols can be confusing [15]. International agreement has specified that natural α-tocopherol should be designated as RRR-α-tocopherol and the synthetic as all-rac-α-tocopherol. In labelling commercial products and in considerable volume of technical literature, however, RRR- forms are designated as d- and all-rac- as dl-.

Commercial Forms of Vitamin E

The common forms of vitamin E used in nutritional supplements and for fortification of foods are:

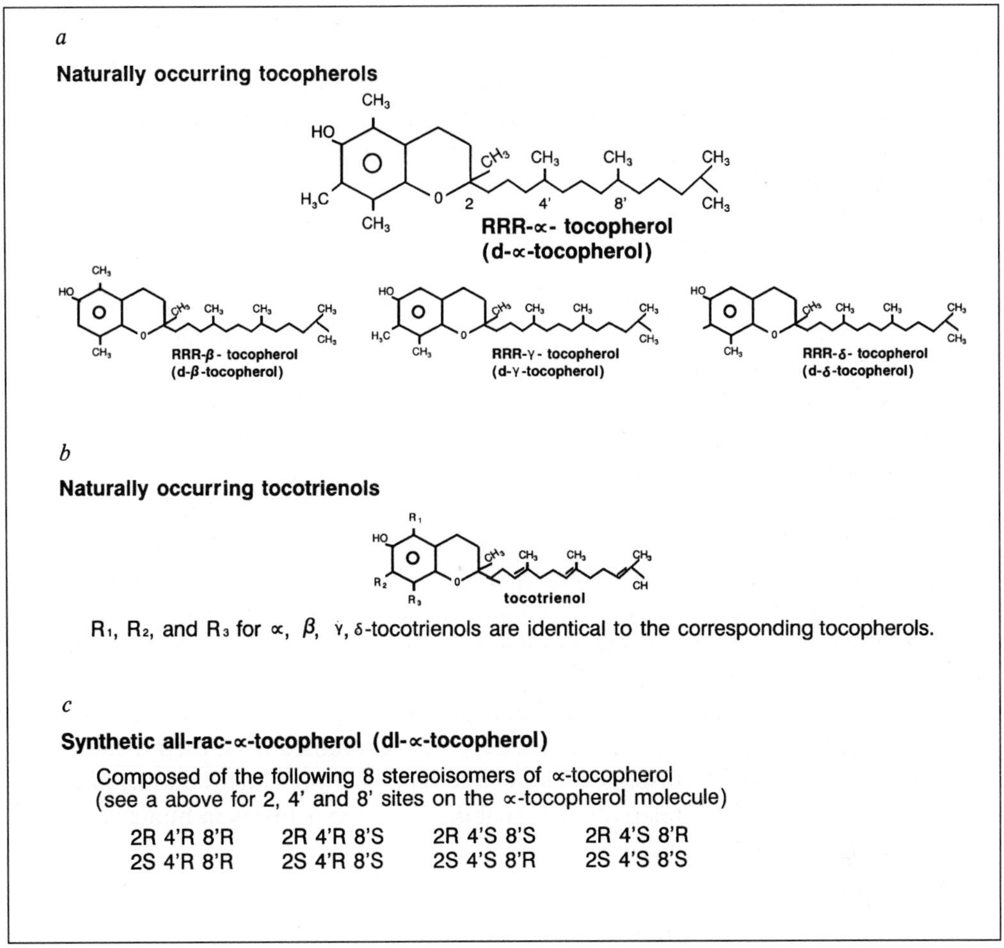

a

Naturally occurring tocopherols

RRR-α- tocopherol
(d-α-tocopherol)

RRR-β- tocopherol
(d-β-tocopherol)

RRR-γ- tocopherol
(d-γ-tocopherol)

RRR-δ- tocopherol
(d-δ-tocopherol)

b

Naturally occurring tocotrienols

tocotrienol

R_1, R_2, and R_3 for α, β, γ, δ-tocotrienols are identical to the corresponding tocopherols.

c

Synthetic all-rac-α-tocopherol (dl-α-tocopherol)

Composed of the following 8 stereoisomers of α-tocopherol
(see a above for 2, 4' and 8' sites on the α-tocopherol molecule)

2R 4'R 8'R	2R 4'R 8'S	2R 4'S 8'S	2R 4'S 8'R
2S 4'R 8'R	2S 4'R 8'S	2S 4'S 8'R	2S 4'S 8'S

Fig. 1. a–c Naturally occurring tocopherols, tocotrienols and stereoisomers of synthetic all-rac-α-tocopherol.

(1) α-Tocopherol, available both in the naturally occurring d- (RRR-) and synthetic dl- (all-rac-) forms.

(2) Esters of α-tocopherol such as acetate and succinate, available both as d- and dl-.

(3) Mixed tocopherols, available mostly in the naturally occurring d-form.

(4) TPGS (d-α-tocopheryl polyethylene glycol 1000 succinate), a water-soluble form.

α-Tocopherol and its acetate and succinate esters are by far the most commonly used forms. Mixed tocopherols are finding increasing, albeit limited use. TPGS is used as the source of vitamin E in some cases of malabsorption.

Biopotency

Understanding the biopotency of vitamin E forms can also be confusing. Biological activity of the major forms was established primarily by the 'fetal resorption-gestation' method in rats, an assay which determines the ability of various forms of vitamin E to maintain live fetuses in pregnant rats; 1.0 mg synthetic all-rac-α-tocopheryl acetate was assigned activity of 1.0 IU and 1.0 mg RRR-α-tocopheryl acetate was assigned 1.36 IU [9, 12]. Biopotencies assigned to other forms of α-tocopherol reflect differences in molecular weight. Recently, the National Research Council (NRC) [15] and others recommended that, for dietary purposes, vitamin E activity be expressed as RRR-α-tocopherol equivalents (α-TE; 1.0 mg RRR-α-tocopherol = 1.0 α-TE; 1.0 mg all-rac-α-tocopherol = 0.74 α-TE). For mixed diets, the NRC proposed the following biopotencies for other natural forms of vitamin E (α-TE/mg): β-tocopherol 0.5; γ-tocopherol 0.1; α-tocotrienol 0.3. Biopotency of esterified forms is computed from their α-tocopherol content. As discussed below, the relative biopotencies do not predict accurately the relative bioavailability of various forms in humans.

Absorption, Transport and Tissue Uptake

α-Tocopherol is absorbed rather inefficiently from the gut into the lymphatic system [6]. Lipases, produced by the pancreas, and bile, produced by the liver, are needed for absorption of fat-soluble forms. Esters such as α-tocopheryl acetate and succinate are first hydrolyzed by lipases to produce α-tocopherol. Bile emulsifies α-tocopherol and forms micelles thus facilitating its absorption. In contrast to the fat-soluble forms, TPGS, a water-soluble form of vitamin E apparently forms micelles and can be absorbed without the need for bile salts [16].

α-Tocopherol is transported from the gut by chylomicrons. During chylomicron catabolism by lipoprotein lipases, a small portion may be transferred to other lipoproteins and tissues. The majority of α-tocopherol reaches the liver by uptake of chylomicron remnants and is then secreted in very low density lipoproteins (VLDL) and transported into the plasma. VLDL is catabolized by lipoprotein lipases into low density lipoproteins (LDL). α-Tocopherol is transferred to high density lipoprotein (HDL) from chylomicrons and LDL, and from VLDL during its catabolism.

Uptake of α-tocopherol by tissues is not understood well. It was suggested that the LDL receptor functions as the mechanism of transport but recent work showed normal tissue levels are maintained even without functional receptors. Transfer of α-tocopherol from HDL to cells and tissues is efficient and occurs without uptake of the whole HDL particle.

Other tocopherols are apparently absorbed and transported in the liver in a similar manner but appear in the blood [6] and tissues at lower concentrations due to a biodiscrimination mechanism dicussed below.

Aspects of Bioavailability and Biokinetics

New Methodology

Significant progress in vitamin E research was made possible by the development of tocopherols labelled with deuterium which can be safely evaluated in humans. Their absorption, transport and uptake in the tissue is measured using gas chromatography-mass spectrometry. This methodology was first developed and used at the National Research Council in Canada [6, 17].

Effect of Chirality

We studied, in cooperation with East Tennessee State University, the biokinetics and relative bioavailability of RRR- and all-rac-α-tocopheryl acetate in six adult humans (3 M, 3 F) ages 25–59 years using isotopes labelled in the 5 (d_3-RRR-) or 5 and 7 (d_6-all-rac-) positions of the chroman ring. Each person received daily for 11 days one capsule containing 150 mg each d_3-RRR- and d_6-all-rac. Blood samples were collected before, during and post dosing and plasma and red blood cells analyzed for d_0-(non-labelled), d_3-, and d_6-α-tocopherol. Results summarized in figure 2, indicate that concentration of RRR- in plasma and red blood cells was substantially higher than all-rac-. Relative bioavailability computed from the area under the concentration curve (RRR/all-rac), was also substan-

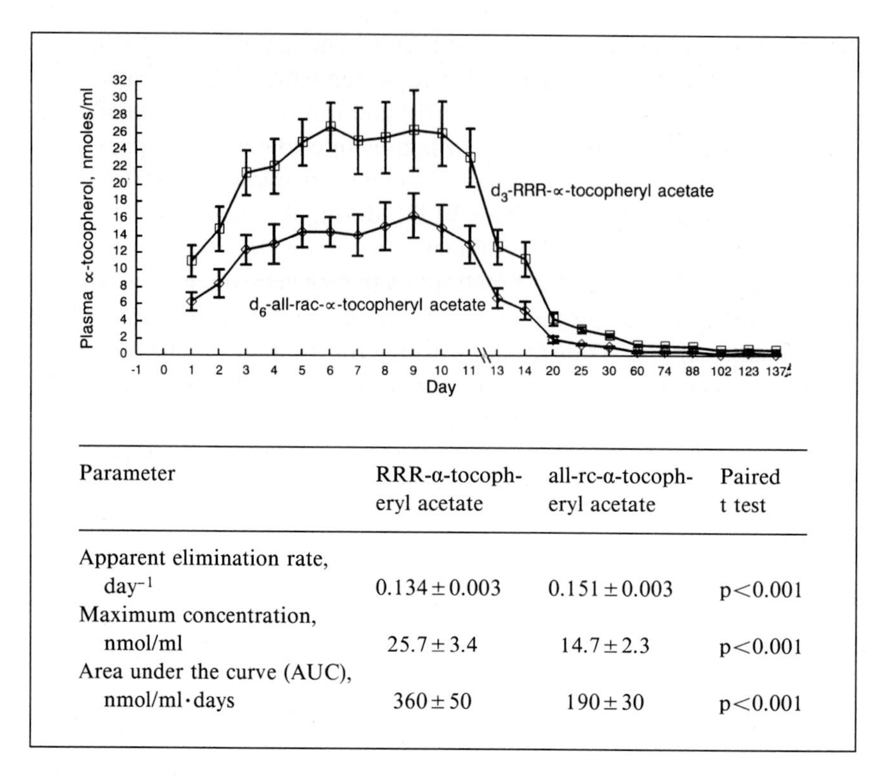

Parameter	RRR-α-tocopheryl acetate	all-rc-α-tocopheryl acetate	Paired t test
Apparent elimination rate, day^{-1}	0.134±0.003	0.151±0.003	$p<0.001$
Maximum concentration, nmol/ml	25.7±3.4	14.7±2.3	$p<0.001$
Area under the curve (AUC), nmol/ml·days	360±50	190±30	$p<0.001$

Fig. 2. Plasma concentration and biokinetic parameters of deuterated RRR-α- and all-rac-α-tocopherol in humans. Six volunteers received orally for 11 days 150 mg/day d_3-RRR- plus 150 mg/day d_6-all-rac-α-tocopheryl-acetate (d_3 and d_6 refer to the number of deuteria on the chroman ring).

tially higher (1.94) than expected from their ratio of biopotencies (1.36). Differences in apparent absorption rates were very small. Although the elimination rate was higher for all-rac- than RRR-, is accounted for only a small part of the observed difference in relative bioavailability. Thus, absorption and elimination could not explain the major differences between RRR- and all-rac.

Other researchers [6, 18] reported similar results and proposed the liver as the site of a major biodiscrimination mechanism favoring RRR-tocopherol. The naturally occurring RRR-α- synthetic stereoisomer SRR-α-tocopherol, given to humans as deuterium-labelled acetate esters, were absorbed without discrimination and secreted into the chylomicrons. The

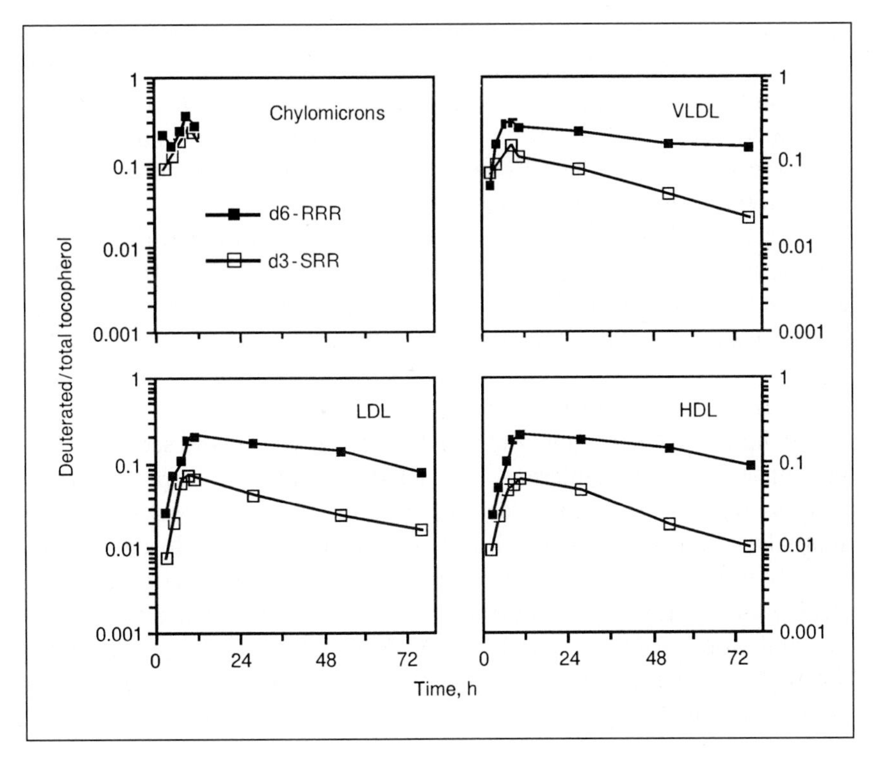

Fig. 3. RRR- and SRR-α-tocopherols are secreted without discrimination in human chylomicrons, but RRR-α-tocopherol is preferentially secreted in very low density lipoproteins. From Traber et al. [19].

RRR-α-tocopherol, however, was preferentially secreted in nascent VLDL in the liver and was the predominant form in LDL and HDL [19] (fig. 3).

Free α-Tocopherol vs. α-Tocopheryl Esters

Tocopherols occur naturally in food in the free (unesterified) form. Commercial vitamin E supplements contain α-tocopherol but more often, its acetate or succinate esters which are more stable. Thus, relative bioavailability of these forms is of practical interest.

Bioavailability of RRR-α-tocopherol and its acetate ester in humans was reported as similar or slightly higher for the free tocopherol form [6].

Relative bioavailability of the RRR- succinate ester appeared lower than for the corresponding acetate and tocopherol forms (unpublished data). The reason for this difference has not been elucidated but it is unlikely to be related to biodiscrimination in the liver since all forms supply RRR-α-tocopherol. Rather, the difference may be due to the rate of hydrolysis and micelle formation in the digestive tract.

TPGS, a water-soluble form, is used as a source of vitamin E for cholestatic children and in some other cases of fat malabsorption [16, 20]. It is also used in some animal species including elephants and black rhinoceros which absorb fat-soluble forms poorly [10, 11].

α-Tocopherol versus Other Tocopherols

In humans, RRR-α and γ-tocopherols are absorbed and secreted from the intestine in chylomicrons, but RRR-α-tocopherol is preferentially incorporated into the VLDL secreted from the liver thus resulting in substantially lower levels in blood and tissues. In monkeys, dosed simultaneously with deuterium labelled RRR-α, SRR-α-tocopheryl acetate and RRR-γ-tocopherol, results indicated similar absorption but a strong biodiscrimination (RRR-α $>$ RRR-γ $>$ SRR-α) in the VLDL secreted in the liver [6]. Limited data suggest similar biodiscrimination favoring α- over β- and δ-tocopherols.

Mechanism of Biodiscrimination

It was suggested that a tocopherol binding protein in the liver was responsible for the biodiscrimination and preferential transfer of RRR-α-tocopherol to VLDL. While crude extracts were prepared earlier [18], it was only recently that this protein was purified from rat livers and characterized [21]. This protein was shown to have strong affinity for α- and β-tocopherols and lower for others. Further research is needed to determine whether a similar liver protein is responsible for biodiscrimination in humans favoring the RRR-α over the all-rac-α-tocopherol.

Tissue Uptake and Depletion

Studies with deuterium-labelled tocopherols, now in progress, will augment the very limited data available on uptake and depletion of tocopherols by various tissues in humans. In rats and guinea pigs, tissue differences were reported in uptake and turnover of tocopherol [6, 17]. Burton and his co-workers [6] classified most tissues as fast (plasma, red blood cells, spleen and liver) or slow (heart, testis, muscle, brain and spinal cord). Indirect evidence from biokinetic modelling of the post-dosing phase in humans, indicated fast and slow disposition rate [unpubl. data]. Strong tissue biodiscrimination (except for liver) was reported [17] in rats favoring the naturally occurring stereoisomer of α-tocopherol (RRR-) over one of the synthetic (SRR-). Other researchers reported a 4- to 6-fold higher accumulation of RRR-α than all-rac-α-tocopherol in rat red blood cells. Biodiscrimination in other tissues was as predicted by their biopotencies [22].

Optimum Intake of Vitamin E

The recommended dietary allowance (RDA) is 10 α-TE for men and 8 for women (15 and 12 IU) [15]. It has been suggested that a significantly higher intake is required for health promotion and disease prevention [23] and in many studies intakes of 100–800 IU were evaluated [23, 24]. Similar high levels were used in many studies on exercise and physical fitness [1, 2, 3, 8]. Further research is needed to determine optimum intake.

Mechanisms of Action

Exercise increases oxygen metabolism and, consequently, production of peroxides and free radicals as evidenced by higher levels of serum malondialdehyde, pentane in breath and other indices [1].

Of major interest is the exercise-induced increase in the mitochondrial content of skeletal muscles which, along with the brain, exhibit the highest oxidative activity of all tissues in humans. At the site of the respiratory chain and fatty acid oxidation, mitochondria and especially their membranes, are exposed to free radicals. A significant increase in mitochondria concentration and respiratory activity while vitamin E remains constant, may increase damage from free radicals [1, 5, 7, 25]. Peroxides and free radicals damage mitochondrial and red blood cell membranes resulting in leakage of enzymes and other proteins. Increased creatine kinase in serum, 3-methylhistidine in urine and other indices signal enzyme leakage. Leakage from muscle cells combined with fatty acid tissue oxidation may cause transient increase in circulating plasma and red blood cell vitamin E [4, 25–27]. Fragility of red blood cells persists following exercise despite increases in their vitamin E and other antioxidant content [4].

As a major lipid-soluble chain-breaking antioxidant in cell membranes, vitamin E reduces production of harmful oxidized products and free radicals. Lipid peroxides and dysfunctional oxidized proteins have adverse effects on health and fitness; oxidized lipoproteins, particularly LDL, have been implicated in atherosclerosis [28, 29]. Vitamin E is essential for maintaining the integrity of cell membranes and thus reduces leakage of enzymes from the muscle and lysis of red blood cells.

The mechanism of action of vitamin E may include the immune system. It was shown recently that heavy exercise induces a series of immune reactions similar to the acute-phase response to infection and tissue injury, including mobilization and activation of neutrophils, proteolysis of skeletal muscle, and increased production of cytokines IL-1b and IL-6 and reduced age-related differences [3, 4]. Vitamin E prevented increase of IL-1b and reduced IL-6. In addition, it enhanced delayed type hypersensitivity, proliferation of Con-A lymphocytes and IL-2 production in elderly indicating a potential to reduce the adverse effects of heavy exercise [24]. Further research is needed to understand the function of vitamin E on the immune system and elucidate other mechanisms.

Conclusions and Practical Applications

Strenuous exercise accelerates the production of free radicals and affects the body's defense system in a similar manner as infection and injury. Vitamin E protects against oxidative damage by reducing production of free radicals and possibly by other mechanisms including the immune system. The following aspects of biokinetics and bioavailability are important in optimizing its effect.

(1) While supplementation increases the blood circulating levels rapidly, uptake by tissues varies significantly and is generally slower. For this reason, supplementation for at least several weeks before strenuous activity is required in order to replete tissues exhibiting slow uptake including muscle and nerve tissue.

(2) A strong biodiscrimination mechanism, probably operating in the liver, affects the utilization and tissue uptake of various tocopherols. Specifically from the naturally occurring tocopherols, RRR-α-tocopherol is preferentially secreted (over γ- and possibly β- and δ-) in blood lipoproteins and is available in higher concentration for uptake by tissues. In addition, RRR-α-tocopherol has been suggested to be preferentially secreted over the synthetic all-rac-α-tocopherol. Tissues may reflect or exceed biodiscrimination observed in the blood. For this reason, the bioavailability of the vitamin E form used is important in obtaining optimum protection.

(3) From the esters of RRR-α-tocopherol, acetate appears to be utilized almost as well as the free tocopherol while utilization of succinate is lower. The water-soluble form TPGS is used by malabsorbers.

(4) The optimum intake of vitamin E for strenuous physical activity and exercise is not known. Because exercise may cause rapid depletion of muscle vitamin E, it has been suggested that higher levels of supplementation are required. In many studies reported to date, intakes many-fold (10–80×) higher than the RDA were evaluated without adverse effects [30]. Immune responses, which appear to be important in reducing adverse effects of strenuous exercise, benefit from such high levels of vitamin E.

References

1 Bendich A: Exercise and free radicals: Effects of antioxidant vitamins; in Brouns F (ed): Advances in Nutrition and Top Sport. Med Sport Sci, vol 32. Basel, Karger, 1991, pp 59–78.
2 Cannon JG, Orencole SF, Fielding RA, et al: Acute phase response in exercise: Interaction of age and vitamin E on neutrofils and muscle enzyme release. Am J Physiol 1990;259:1214–1219.
3 Cannon JG, Meydani SN, Fielding RA, et al: Acute phase response in exercise. II. Assocations between vitamin E, cytokines and muscle proteolysis. Am J Physiol 1990;260:1235–1240.
4 Duthie GG, Robertson JD, Maughan RJ, Morice PC: Blood antioxidant status and erythrocyte peroxidation following distance running. Arch Biochem Biophys 1990; 282:78–83.
5 Packer L, Almada AL, Rothfuss LM, Wilson DS: Modulation of tissue vitamin E levels by physical exercise; in Diplock AT, et al (eds): Biochemistry and Health Implications. Ann NY Acad Sci 1990;57:311–321.
6 Burton GW, Traber MG: Vitamin E: Antioxidant activity, biokinetics and bioavailability. Ann Rev Nutr 1990;10:357–382.
7 Sumida S, Tanaka K, Kitao K, et al: Exercise induced lipid peroxidation and leakage of enzymes before and after vitamin E supplementation. Int J Biochem 1989;21: 835–838.
8 Simon-Schnass I, Pabst H: Influence of vitamin E on physical performance. Int J Vitam Nutr Res 1988;58:49–54.
9 Desai ID: Assay methods; in Machlin LJ (ed): Vitamin E: A Comprehensive Treatise. New York, Marcel Dekker, 1980, pp 67–98.
10 Papas AM, Acuff RV, Hidiroglou N, et al: Comparative bioavailability of vitamin E in animals and humans: Effect of chemical form, solubility and chirality. Intern. Sympos. Vit E. Kawashima, Gifu, September 1991.
11 Papas AM, Cambre RC, Citino SB, Sokol RJ: Efficacy of absorption of various forms of vitamin E by captive elephants and black rhinoceros. J Zoo Wildlife Med 1991;22:309–317.

12 Herting DC: Vitamin E, in the Kirk-Othmer: Encyclopedia of Chemical Technology. New York, 1984, vol 24, pp 214–227.
13 Diplock AT (ed): Vitamin E, in Fat-Soluble Vitamins: Their Biochemistry and Applications. Lancaster, Pennsylvania Technomic Publications, 1985.
14 Bauernfeind J: Tocopherols in foods; in Machlin LJ (ed): Vitamin E: A Comprehensive Treatise. New York, Marcel Dekker, 1980, pp 99–167.
15 NRC (National Research Council): Recommended Dietary Allowances, ed. 10. Washington, National Academy of Sciences, 1989.
16 Traber MG, Kayden HJ, Green JB, Green MH: Absorption of water-miscible forms of vitamin E in a patient with cholestasis and in thoracic duct-cannulated rats. Am J Clin Nutr 1986;44:914–923.
17 Ingold KU, Burton GW, Foster DO, et al: Biokinetics of and discrimination between dietary RRR- and SRR-α-tocopherols in the male rat. Lipids 1987;22:163–172.
18 Catignani GL, Bieri JG: Rat liver α-tocopherol binding protein. Biochim Biophys Acta 1977;497:349–357.
19 Traber MG, Burton GW, Ingold KU, Kayden HJ: RRR- and SRR-α-tocopherols are secreted without discrimination in human chylomicrons, but RRR-α-tocopherol is preferentially secreted in very low density lipoproteins. J Lipid Res 1990;31:675–685.
20 Sokol RJ, Butler-Simon N, Heubi JE, et al: Vitamin E deficiency neuropathy in children with fat malabsorption. Studies in cystic fibrosis and chronic cholestasis. Ann NY Acad Sci 1989;570:156–168.
21 Sato Y, Hagiwara K, Arai H, Inoue K: Purification and characterization of the α-tocopherol transfer protein from rat liver. FEBS Lett 1991;288:41–45.
22 Behrens WA, Madere R: Tissue biodiscrimination between dietary RRR-α- and all-rac-α-tocopherol in rats. J Nutr 1991;121:454–459.
23 Horwitt MK: Data supporting supplementation of humans with vitamin E. J Nutr 1991;121:424–429.
24 Meydani SN, Barklund MP, Liu S, et al: Vitamin E supplementation enhances cell-mediated immunity in healthy elderly subjects. Am J Clin Nutr 1990;52:557–563.
25 Bowles DK, Torgan CE, Ebner S, et al: Effects of accute, submaximal exercise on skeletal muscle vitamin E. Free Radic Res Commun 1991;14:139–143.
26 Robertson JD, Maughan RJ, Duthie GG, Morrice PC: Increased blood antioxidant systems of runners in response to training load. Clin Sci 1991;80:611–618.
27 Rokitzki L, Porath B, Schmidt S, et al: Changes in the concentrations of vitamin E, lipoprotein and free fatty acid glycerides after a marathon race. Fett Wiss Technol 1990;92:331–334.
28 Esterbauer H, Dieber-Rotheneder M, Waeg G, et al: Biochemical, structural, and functional properties of oxidized low-density lipoprotein. Chem Res Toxicol 1990; 3:77–92.
29 Steinberg D: Antioxidants and atherosclerosis: A current assessment. Circulation 1991;84:1420–1425.
30 Bendich A, Machlin LJ: Safety of oral intake of vitamin E. Am J Clin Nutr 1988;48: 612–619.

Andreas M. Papas, PhD, Eastman Chemical Company, PO Box 1974,
Kingsport, TN 37662 (USA)

Simopoulos AP (ed): Nutrition and Fitness in Health and Disease.
World Rev Nutr Diet. Basel, Karger, 1993, vol 72, pp 177–189

Nutrition and Fitness Recommendations When Science is in Transition

Vitamin and Mineral Supplementation: A Case in Point

Steven M. Zifferblatt

Better Life Institute, Grand Rapids, Mich., USA

'These are the times that try men's souls' said Thomas Paine, American Revolutionary War Patriot and author of the pamphlet 'Common Sense'. Mr. Paine was referring to the hardships the American Colonies faced when they decided to undertake their War of Independence in 1776. Today, in 1992, 'these are the times that try our souls'. We are facing an extraordinary challenge and opportunity to extend man's length and quality of life far beyond the century old four score and five years. The sciences underlying nutrition and fitness will likely play a major role.

The Ultimate Challenge: Science

As we approach the 21st century we will progress beyond mid-century science and medicine that employed a disease, drug and surgical model to extend man's life. Despite our current life expectancy of 85 years, man's biological life span is between 110 and 120 years. With the coming age of molecular, cellular and genetic medicine the secrets of the life of a single cell will be unlocked and man's life will be extended far beyond the limitations governed by today's medicine and life-style.

The Practical Challenge: Health Recommendations

But the challenge to extend and improve life is more than that of progress in science and medicine. It is also a challenge to improve its application in daily life. This is the subject of this paper. As we strive to improve the science behind nutrition and fitness we also need to make an equal effort to improve its application and integration in everyday life. The current health recommendations regarding vitamins and minerals for prevention of disease and health promotion will be discussed as a case in point.

The public, for example, lacks information from the government about the pros and cons of use of antioxidant vitamins and n–3 fatty acid food supplements [1–3]. Contradictory recommendations exist between regulatory agencies (US Food and Drug Administration, FDA), research institutes (National Cancer Institute, NIH), and the Centers for Disease Control (CDC) [4–6]. The public is entitled to *all* the facts – what we know, do not know, likely will know and pros and cons. They then can make their own decision. The challenge is less to tell the public what to do and more to educate and inform them of the dynamic and increasing potential of proper use of food supplements.

The transfer of scientific and medical knowledge to health recommendations starts with government and institutional consensus regarding the status of science and technology in question. These recommendations are formalized and the proceedings published and made available to be public. For the most part, it has worked well. There are four 'gatekeepers' by which medical information is provided to the public: (1) basic research science and medicine consensus recommendations; (2) the mass media; (3) the practicing physician, and (4) business: the food and health product industry.

But our present transfer system does not seem to work well in the area of nutrition and fitness. The supportive science is still in transition and rapidly growing. Many of our current health recommendations are too static, conservative or vague. The information and health recommendations communicated to the public can be inconsistent, often contradictory and not representative of up-to-date data [4–6].

A recent commentary by Willet [7] on the importance of folic acid supplementation to prevent neural tube defects is an excellent example of how a conservative, static approach by the FDA does not serve the public interest very well. '... The present body of evidence (folic acid supplementation) provides an excellent example of how data from observational epidemiologic and randomized trials can be most informative when viewed as complementary ... The Food and Drug Administration is proposing that the effect of folic acid on risk of neural tube defects not be allowed as a health claim and that the US RDA of 0.4 mg/day be reduced to 0.18

mg/day. The unwillingness of official US agencies to generalize even slightly from the conditions of the Medical Research Council study is most disturbing ...'

Willet [7] goes on to point out that evidence supporting folic acid supplementation is much stronger than that supporting reducing saturated fat intake to reduce risk of heart disease. Finally, Willet points out that definitive data is unlikely to be forthcoming and we need to decide with current available data. '... Because a randomized placebo-controlled trial of periconceptional folic acid supplementation ... would almost surely be considered unethical, further directly relevant experimental data are unlikely to become available ...'

Are the interest of our perinatal women being served well by the reluctance of the FDA to leap beyond its current policy of no supplementation unless proved beyond a shadow of a doubt? ... probably not!

Guidance on many important nutrition and fitness issues today can be inconsistent and vague; medical, surgical, nutrition and exercise management of heart disease, frequency and intensity of general aerobic exercise, postmenopausal hormone supplementation, effective and safe methods for weight control, effective cosmetic skin care, childhood nutrition and exercise to prevent adult degenerative diseases, vitamin and mineral supplementation, sports and muscle-building food supplements and the safety of artificial sweeteners, food additives and food irradiation.

The public's confusion is partly understandable. If nutrition and fitness data are not definitive, no definitive recommendations can be offered. Interpretation and judgement is then provided by the four 'gatekeepers': science, media, practitioner and business. But, each has a different perspective and the public receives health recommendations that can be vague, inconsistent, contradictory and, finally, confusing. A new model is required to meet modern health challenges in the area of nutrition and fitness when the underlying science is in transition – incomplete and rapidly developing. We need to use these four gatekeepers for health recommendations more constructively for the following reasons.

Scientific Knowledge Progression

The rate at which science advances today is unprecedented. As new recommendations are being discussed, new advances in related research are being made. At this very moment, as we discuss the importance of dietary reductions in saturated fat [1–3], new data on lipid transport, fatty acids [8], lipid-lowering drugs, genetic enzymatic defects [9] are challenging these recommendations. The public reads about these new developments, but lacks specific uniform, fluid and practical guidance.

Information Dissemination

The rate at which scientific information is disseminated to the public is extremely rapid – almost instantaneous. The speed and multiplicity of sources through which new information proliferates is increasing. Discussions of data presented at scientific conferences and meetings are commonplace in daily media. Books, magazines, radio and talk shows on medicine and health are at 'epidemic' level. Equally important, the information conveyed appears to be authoritative, but is often based on judgement and advocacy, sometimes professional, often lay.

Delivery of Medical Care

The traditional treatment centered, and paternalistic role (protect the public from itself) in the area of nutrition and fitness is becoming outdated: (1) a better-informed consumer seeks more participation in the doctor-patient relationship, and (2) increased emphasis on life-style changes; nutrition and exercise place treatment in hands other than those of the physician.

Nutrition and Fitness are 'Big Business'

Nutrition and fitness has become an economic arena in which many players compete for the public's attention and pocketbook. Aside from traditional health professionals, others, specifically, gourmet chef, herbalist, aerobic instructor, franchised health program, health food companies, celebrities and countless books and magazines, now compete successfully with medicine and science for the attention of the public. Health recommendations are no longer solely governed by science and medicine. New and changing knowledge, rate and means of information dissemination, philosophies of health care and marketplace dynamics have challenged this century-old process. Need, speed, creed and greed have changed it forever – indeed!

'These are the times that try men's souls' – the souls of scientist, publisher, physician and businessman alike. The public is not getting the guidance it needs. We do not yet enlist the best qualities, best of all these four factors: science, information dissemination, medical care and business and apply them to the health challenges of modern life. The nutrition and fitness concerns of the public need to be better served. We should consider a different and fresh approach to the challenge of technology transfer. There are some precedents.

The NHLBI (NIH) Model and the Cholesterol Controversy

In 1977, the National Heart, Lung and Blood Institute launched a pilot cholesterol and fat nutrition education program in 116 supermarkets in the Washington, DC-Baltimore area. At that time NHLBI was sponsoring or coordinating numerous clinical trials directed at the cholesterol hypothesis, from basic research to demonstration studies. NHLBI wished to avoid any definitive dietary recommendation about cholesterol and saturated fat prior to the results of the research programs, but the public was confused. Ideally, NHLBI would have preferred to wait until the studies were completed. But heart disease was at epidemic proportions and the public wanted definitive nutrition guidance. The situation facing NHLBI and the four gatekeepers was 'very dynamic'.

Research at many levels of scientific inference demonstrated a relationship between dietary saturated fat, serum cholesterol and cardiovascular disease. At the same time lipid transport research was emerging as a key factor. Simultaneously, enzyme and genetic research was minimizing lifestyle factors [8].

Scientific and medical consensus committees – NHLBI, National Academy of Sciences, the American Heart Association, the American Health Foundation, and the World Health Organization – were inconsistent or vague in their recommendations to the public. Stanford, Minnesota, Pennsylvania and UCLA Medical Schools recommended 'that dietary changes were necessary'. Finland was actively discouraging consumption of whole milk dairy products while Britain was encouraging it.

Numerous articles, books, pamphlets, radio and television presentations started to emerge. Consumer advocate organizations such as The

Center for Science in the Public Interest implied a conspiracy existed. Consumer organizations lobbied Congress to pressure NHLBI to provide more definitive proactive health recommendations [10–13]. The meat, dairy and cereal industry published 'nutrition information' literature that was contradictory regarding need for dietary change. Stanford, the University of California at Los Angeles and Minnesota Medical Schools were involved in research on nutrition education and behavior change, tantamount to actual health care. Other scientists publicly minimized cholesterol's importance. The media sensationalized and scapegoats were encouraged ... it was 'dirty'! At the same time the American Medical Association and the American Dietary Association adopted a disease oriented conservative 'wait and see', or 'talk to your doctor' policy. Other allied health professions jumped into the void. Dentists and chriopractors, exercise physiologists and fitness instructors became advocates of changes in nutrition and exercise habits. Corporations such as Xerox, Johnson & Johnson and Control Data invested tens of millions in employee nutrition and exercise-based nutrition and wellness programs. Patients sought help elsewhere than their doctor's office or hospital clinic.

Numerous products proliferated the marketplace. The age of 'nutritious' foods, food supplements, sports drinks, over the counter drugs, liquid diets, pills, spas and risk reduction centers and exercise equipment was born. Everything had 'no cholesterol' in it and on it! Major corporations purchased health food companies and good health became good business.

Today the health business is one of the fastest-growing markets in the United States. It will likely expand in a similar way to all Western nations. The result was 'nutrition and fitness information dysfunction'. The best qualities of the four gatekeepers were not provided to the public. Scientists were polarized, media senstationalized and made scapegoats, physicians discouraged patient dialogue and became authoritative, and business overextended product health claims [14, 15].

In the face of this controversy, the NHLBI launched a pilot consumer cholesterol nutrition education program 'Foods for Health' in the supermarket [16]. Giant Foods, a pioneer and leader in consumer education cooperated with NHLBI. The purpose of this research program was to demonstrate the feasibility of educating the public at the 'point of decision'. If the program was successful this would be a proven model for delivering nutrition information at the point of purchase. But more important and central to the point of this paper the NHLBI departed from convention in the manner they presented nutritional information to the shopper. The nation's basic biomedical research institution publicly recognized the controversy, the need and the fluidity of cholesterol research and provided the public a dialogue format for health decisions and specifically recommended that each person think and decide for themselves.

The Basic Theme of the Program Was 'You Decide'

The 'You Decide' supermarket nutrition education program provided bi-weekly six-page 'Eater's Almanacs' and graphic educational food product signs, 'Shelf Talkers' in 116 supermarkets. Each brochure contained recipes, graphics and information written at the sixth grade educational level. The information contained in this program was reviewed by a team of NHLBI physicians, research scientists, nutritionists and educators and followed the guidelines below:

(1) Heart disease and nutrition relationships were discussed.

(2) The transitional state of the science was acknowledged.

(3) The present scientific facts as NHLBI knew them were presented ... what we knew, or did not know, what were the risks and benefits.

(4) Each Eater's Almanac and Shelf Talker specifically said to each consumer 'You Decide'.

NHLBI assumed a unique role during these 'transitional times'. NHLBI (1) explicitly acknowledged the lack of definitive data; (2) provided the public with objective information, recognized the controversy, and (3) asked the public to decide on these matters for themselves.

A similar model should be considered for nutrition and fitness. It should have the following capabilities:

(1) Recognize and legitimize the fluidity and complexity of scientific data.

(2) Outline the available alternatives: medical, surgical and lifestyle.

(3) Discuss the pros and cons of these alternatives from a risk-benefit and cost-benefit perspective.

(4) Offer guidance but explicitly ask the public to use their intelligence and common sense to decide for themselves.

(5) Continually inform and update the public and ask them to update their personal decisions.

This is the type of fluid inferential model we require in today's transitional times – a form that is educational and continually encourages and guides each person's use of their intellect and common sense. Daily vitamin and mineral supplementation is a case in point.

'To Supplement ... or Not To Supplement'

Each day about 100 million Americans, young and old, rich and poor, educated and uneducated, peoples of all races eat one or more food supplements (vitamin and mineral tablets, capsules, food concentrates and liquids) [17, 18]. Major American and international pharmaceutical corporations produce and/or retail vitamin and mineral supplements. Major food companies produce fortified foods. Food supplement sales exceed $ 3 billion yearly. Yet this health habit is actively discouraged at governmental, institutional and medical practice levels [19, 20]; a significant discrepancy with the actions of the public. The public is in the middle of this dysfunction. It is confused and lacks proper guidance. The gatekeepers are not integrated or serving the public very well.

Scientific and medical research is continually reporting new findings relating to the potential of certain vitamins and minerals to prevent and treat degenerative disease such as heart disease, cancer, arthritis, cataracts and osteoporosis [21]. The recommendation emanating from the government and institutions is a static 'do nothing unless there is a diagnosed medical reason', usually a disease related to a documented nutritional deficiency, for using food supplements. Mass media continually seeks and reports these findings. They provide lay and expert, but subjectively and selectively reviewed commentaries. Opinion, advocacy and sensationalism are often employed to compete for the public's attention [22]. Patients seeking recommendations and personal guidance from their physicians and dieticians on navigating these confusing waters are often met with a flat 'no' or an emotional 'I don't care and don't waste your money', or 'it can hurt you' statement (somewhat similar to the dietary recommendations offered 7 years ago about fat, fiber and cholesterol when the 'You Decide' program was completed). Some physicians recommend food supplements for general prevention purposes under certain biological conditions: pregnancy, early infancy, the elderly, and during weight loss. Vitamin and mineral and specifically fortified food sales are increasing. Corporate backed special interest magazines, advertisements, 'advertorials' and suggestive labeling encourage aggressive buying habits among a health sensitive public.

Vitamin and Mineral Supplementation: The Science

Within the last 3 years numerous articles relating food supplements to either the prevention or treatment of degenerative disease have been published in peer-reviewed scientific and medical journals [21, 23]. For example, many conferences on cellular oxidation processes, immunoincompetence, inflammatory disease and metabolic deficits in the aging population centered on the potential role and benefits of vitamin and mineral supplementation have been held in the United States, Britain and Japan. Some scientists have concluded it is difficult, if not impossible, to achieve optimum nutrition by merely relying upon daily meals and the manner in which produce is supplied [24].

The Risk Benefits

The data accumulated indicates few side effects or adverse health consequences exist with the rational and regular use of food supplements [21]. Reports on the side effects due to excess dosage are extremely rare, mainly reversible and attributed to extremely irrational use. The potential for benefit is significant, especially in view of the fact that medicine does not yet have effective means to prevent or treat degenerative diseases and many drugs have serious side effects.

The Cost Benefits and Feasibility

Health care costs are increasing at 10–15% per annum. Cost-risk-benefit health care issues are a critical concern in all Western nations. Current therapies to treat degenerative disease are escalating in cost at a fatal economic rate. Many people in the United States, about 30%, do not have health insurance and cannot get it or afford it. The potential for proper use of food supplements to prevent, delay or treat many degenerative diseases exists. Its costs are low. Its availability is universal. Everyone knows how to take tablets, capsules, liquids and powders. Means of dispersal and delivery are in place. This is what we call in the United States a 'no brainer'.

Nutrition and food supplement science portend benefit, economy and feasibility in application with no risk. Food is no longer just something you eat to enjoy and survive. It has an impact on our health. Food is medicine! The public, intuitively, is recognizing this as well. That is the reason use of food supplements is increasing.

Several years ago a major nutrition scientist was asked why he publicly discouraged people against using food supplements while he privately supplemented with vitamins E, C and beta-carotene. He said he understood the subtleties of research trends, potential benefits and risks in relation to his life-style. But it was too difficult to educate the public similarly and therefore he must advise against their use. We must disagree. It may be more difficult. But, it is not impossible, or responsible. This is not a call to abandon regulation and guidance from government and medical institutions. But, times have changed and new ideas are needed. The science related to food supplementation and to the larger body of nutrition and fitness is growing and changing every day. It is impossible to provide definitive recommendations. But, it is possible to offer objective guidance to the public and let them continually decide for themselves on such 'transitional health matters'.

Help the Public Decide for Themselves

We need a fluid, less-paternalistic model – one that recognizes that different health challenges, science, social and economic conditions exist today. The NHLBI 'You Decide' nutrition education program offers a fluid objective and socially responsive model. The NHLBI endorsed a 'You Decide' program for cholesterol education in 1977. There is a precedent for using this same model today for educating the public about vitamins and minerals and their potential to improve health and fight certain diseases. Whether the subject is antioxidants or other highly promising supplements such as n–3 fatty acids it is time to provide the public with an ongoing information base to decide for themselves.

Widespread Use of Food Supplements Might Lead to Medical Economic Catastrophe

Why is such an obvious and rational model not used to objectively provide the public with information on antioxidant and n–3 food supplements? The answer to this question lies in its impact on the economics of medical practice and prescription drug use and development. It does not reside in the FDA or the medical community's concern about the safety or lack of efficacy data of such supplements. If these supplements prevented, delayed or avoided use of more expensive medical and surgical procedures in the slightest degree, the economic impact on physicians, hospitals, drug companies and the fish industry would be catastrophic. This is a political and economic conflict – not a scientific conflict. It is the public that loses the potential of improved health with less discomfort and expense.

The public will always look to and rely upon our government and medical institutions for facts, guidance and objective discussion about science and medicine. But they need better participation in health decisions and the guidance of science and medicine as they decide for themselves. The public is now challenging regulations regarding access to new unproven therapies. Patients and their families question the right of the US Food and Drug Administration to withhold experimental drugs for treating Alzheimer's diseases and AIDS when no effective alternatives exist. People want the government to provide them with the facts as they now stand – pro and con and let them make their own decision. Congress has asked the NIH to review unconventional medical practices [25].

In the final analysis, the health, political, economic and social strength of a society rests upon the availability of objective information and the opportunity for each person to intelligently exercise their right of choice. Science is a method, albeit a powerful one, to help us know things more objectively. But the responsibility of science is more than providing objective information. It is guiding the public in its intelligent use. But we must guide intelligently – not dictate or default to lay forces. To paraphrase Shakespeare, perhaps 'we now guide too well, but not too wisely'. Thomas Paine is still right: 'These are the times that try men's souls', scientist and citizen alike. Help the people decide for themselves!

References

1 US Department of Agriculture, US Department of Health and Human Services: Nutrition and Your Health: Dietary Guidelines for Americans. Home and Garden Bulletin No 232, ed 1. Washington, US Government Printing Office, 1980.
2 US Department of Agriculture, US Department of Health and Human Services: Nutrition and Your Health: Dietary Guidelines for Americans. Home and Garden Bulletin No 232, ed 2. Washington, US Government Printing Office, 1985.
3 US Department of Agriculture, US Department of Health and Human Services:

Nutrition and Your Health: Dietary Guidelines for Americans. Home and Garden Bulletin No 232, ed 3. Washington, US Government Printing Office, 1990.
4 Food and Drug Administration: Food labeling: Health claims and label statements; folic acid and neural tube defects (Docket No 91N-0100); and proposed rulings on the RDI for folic acid (Docket No 90N-0134). Federal Register. November 27, 1991.
5 Butrum RR, Clifford CK, Lanza E: NCI Dietary Guidelines: Rationale. Am J Clin Nutr 1988;48(suppl).
6 Centers for Disease Control: Folic Acid to Prevent Spina Bifida and Other Neural Tube Defects: Meeting (Docket No 92-15398) Federal Register. July 1, 1992; 57(127):29323.
7 Willett WC: Folic acid and neural tube defect: Can't we come to closure? Am J Publ Health 1992;82:666–668.
8 Simopoulos AP, Kifer RR, Martin RE, Barlow SM (ed): Health Effects of w3 polyunsaturated fatty acids in seafoods. World Rev Nutr Diet. Basel, Karger, 1991, vol 66.
9 Simopoulos AP, Childs B (eds): Genetics Variation and Nutrition. World Rev Nutr Diet. Basel, Karger, 1990, vol 63.
10 US Senate Select Committee on Nutrition and Human Needs: The Role of the Federal Government in Human Nutrition Research. Washington, US Government Printing Office, 1976.
11 US Senate Select Committee on Nutrition and Human Needs: Final Report. Washington, US Government Printing Office, 1977.
12 US Senate Select Committee on Nutrition and Human Needs: Dietary Goals for the United States. Washington, US Government Printing Office, 1977.
13 US Senate Select Committee on Nutrition and Human Needs: Dietary Goals for the United States, ed. 2. Washington, US Government Printing Office, 1977.
14 US Public Health Service, US Department of Health and Human Services: Surgeon General's Report on Nutrition and Health. Washington, US Government Printing Office, 1988, publ No [DHHS-PHS] 88-50210.
15 US Public Health Service, US Department of Health and Human Services: Dietary Fads and Frauds, Chap 19. Surgeon General's Report on Nutrition and Health. Washington, US Government Printing Office, 1988, publ No [DHHS-PHS] 88-50210, pp 695-712.
16 Ernst ND, Zifferblatt SM, et al: Nutrition education at the point of purchase: 'The foods for health' project evaluated. Prev Med 1986;15:60–73.
17 Subar AF, Block G: Use of vitamin and mineral supplements: Demographics and amounts of nutrients consumed. The 1987 health interview survey. Am J Epidemiol 1990;132:1091–1101.
18 Food and Drug Administration: Public Meeting: Dietary Supplements [Docket No 91N-0256]. Federal Register. July 16, 1991;56:32436–32437.
19 National Cholesterol Education Program: Report of the National Cholesterol Education Program Expert Panel on Detection, Evaluation and Treatment of High Blood Cholesterol in Adults. Arch Intern Med 1988;148:36–69.
20 Diet and Health: Implications for reducing chronic disease risk. Committee on Diet and Health, Food and Nutrition Board. Washington, Commission on Life Sciences, National Research Council, 1989.

21 Slater TF, Block G (eds): Proceedings of the Conference on Antioxidant Vitamins and Beta-Carotene in Disease Prevention. Am J Clin Nutr 1991;53:189S–396S.
22 Grinell S: RDA for Science; in Simopoulos AP, Childs B (eds): Genetic Variation and Nutrition. World Rev Nutr Diet. Basel, Karger, 1990, vol 63, pp 287–294.
23 Simopoulos AP: Omega-3 fatty acids in health and disease and in growth and development. Am J Clin Nur 1991;54:438–463.
24 Tufts Nutrition Newsletter 1991;9:2.
25 Bryant J: National Institutes of Health. NIH panel reviews 'unconventional' medical practices. The NIH Record. July 7, vol XLIV No 14. Washington, US Government Printing Office, 1992.

Steven M. Zifferblatt, PhD, Better Life Institute, 220 Lyon, Suite 100,
Grand Rapids, MI 49305 (USA)

Panel VII
Update on Policies and Programs in Nutrition and Physical Fitness

Simopoulos AP (ed): Nutrition and Fitness in Health and Disease.
World Rev Nutr Diet. Basel, Karger, 1993, vol 72, pp 190–199

Policies and Programs in Nutrition and Physical Fitness in Central and South America

Eleazar Lara-Pantin

Unidad de Investigaciones en Nutricion, Valencia, Venezuela

When we met here in Greece 4 years ago, I came to talk about the Policies and Programs in Nutrition and Physical Fitness in Venezuela, and I said [1]: 'Venezuela, like many other developing countries, has not yet implemented national or official nutrition and fitness programs and policies aimed at contributing to the health of the population.' Today, I am addressing the same issue in the Central and South American context and I must say that, apart from new socioeconomic elements, such a statement can also be applied to the situation everywhere; the lack of policies and coordinated programs regarding nutrition and fitness is still the common denominator in all the countries of this area.

Everywhere, programs and activities consider mostly the groups practicing sports, leaving aside the growing concern of the larger sector of the population for fitness through noncompetitive exercises.

For decades, one of the characteristics of developing countries has been the lack of policies in all fields. If one evaluates key areas that are meant to support the development process in every country of the region, one will find that, with very few exceptions in some specific areas, the dynamics of agriculture, economics, health and many other fields, is determined by the situation observed at a given moment and not by true national coordinated development programs and policies.

If this is the case with the so-called most important areas, it is easy to imagine what happens with the activities of nutrition and fitness. Underestimation, improvisation and lack of coordination best define the overall situation.

Underestimation and improvisation characterize higher decision levels. Lack of coordination counteracts worthy initiatives carried out in isolation. In summary, as Kihumbu Thairu [2] said in the 1st International Conference on Nutrition and Fitness (ICNF): 'After school, physical fitness is an individual matter.'

Abraham Horwitz [3], former Director of the Pan American Health Organization, said in the inaugural speech of the 1st Symposium of Cavendes Foundation: 'We, in the developing Americas, have distinguished ourselves by the irrational use of the human, material and financial resources when trying to solve social problems. We tend more to dissociate than to coordinate ourselves.'

However, a lack of policies does not mean a lack of action. A lot of individual and institutional sound efforts are in progress, usually not coordinated, as it has been said, but all of them awaiting the decision makers to define policies that would integrate them into organized programs, according to the reality of each country.

Parallel to the negative trends represented by the absence of official policies, a most positive attitude is also common in the whole region; a growing motivation of the population for different forms of exercise, usually associated with an increasing concern for good nutrition. In Central and South America, the same as in developed countries, many people acknowledge nutrition and exercise as important for a healthy life. From Mexico to Argentina, in most sectors of the population, with some variations according to the percentages of people living in urban areas, the importance of nutrition and fitness seems to be a widely accepted concept.

Some countries still have large sectors of their population living in rural areas. Their life is so active that no motivation is needed, or policies required, to encourage people to exercise. For those who eat healthily, walking long distances and working hard in an uncontaminated environment compensates for the unquestionable need to exercise that worries those of us living under the sedentary effects of an urban life.

For the large group of peasants who cannot satisfy their nutritional needs, fitness is not a final product of such an active life.

Although studies made in different countries have shown that, between certain limits of nutritional deficit, the human body tends to remain in energy balance, this is easily broken when people are required to increase the demand through strenuous physical efforts. Sometimes, this is observed when people work harder encouraged by economic incentives [4].

Other times, public health problems are the cause of the energy imbalance. Parasites, bacterial infections and inadequate food patterns and their consequences, seriously limit the above-mentioned theoretical benefits of rural life on fitness; especially when food shortage is accompanied by poor sanitation.

In the highly urbanized areas, motivation about the importance of nutrition and fitness is not enough for most people. Each one of the Central and South American countries is suffering, in various degrees of severity, the impact of the economic crisis produced by the implementation of a common strategy promoted to make them able to pay their external debts to common creditors.

Strangely enough, countries traditionally unable to develop rational economic and agricultural policies in line with their own realities, have been able to follow literally those suggested and forced by international financing agencies, regardless of their negative impact on the lower sectors of the population. Moreover, this 'conflicting by-product', the deterioration of life conditions and, consequently, of the nutritional status of the majority of the population, although difficult to accept, seems to be an expected consequence of such policies [5].

This reality directly confronts the principle stated by Phillipe Stroot [6], the WHO Representative to the 1st ICNF: 'In developing countries, governments have to balance, not only their budgets, but also their diet and food policies.'

Seven years ago, when discussing the problem of obesity in developing countries, I wrote [7]: 'When we talk about developing countries we mean people who are improving their general situation, i.e. moving up the scale of social mobility which does not necessarily mean getting better in every aspect of life.' Now, after the 'lost decade' many things have changed a great deal for us, and most of them are looking worse. Important sectors of the population living in Central and South American countries are now moving down the scale of social mobility, and poverty is increasing its prevalence in a dramatic way.

In an interesting paper devoted to the debt crisis in Latin America, Jackie Roddick [9] tells the following about the Bolivian miners' situation:

'In line with traditional International Monetary Fund (IMF) policies, government subsidies to consumers were cut back drastically. Freed from such subsidies, the price of bread rose fourfold. As the state gas and oil companies began to charge 'economic prices' to consumers, the price of a bottle of domestic gas went up twenty times, a liter of petrol seven times. At the same time, wages were frozen below the rate of inflation .... Measures had savage consequences for the 80% of Bolivians whom the International Labour Office (ILO) estimates to be living in absolute poverty, as it triggered a drastic rise in their living costs. Latin America has been squeezed between burgeoning debt payments and shrinking export revenues, in a classic scissors crisis. In a decade notable for the self righteousness of Latin America's creditors, the plight of the Bolivian miners mirrors the fate of the majority of Latin America's poor. The region has been earning less and less for its exports, not just in terms of their prices in world markets, but also in terms of what the revenue from them can purchase in manufactured goods – what economists call their "terms of trade".'

A good example of the adequacy of that final statement can be found in the Venezuelan situation. Besides being an oil producing and exporting country, around 80% of the population also qualifies as poor [9]; perhaps with a lower degree of poverty than Bolivians, but poor enough as to see their body iron stores depleted in such a way that prevalence of low ferritin levels in students between 7 and 15 years of age increased by 80% in 5 years [Layrisse, personal commun.]. Obviously, learning possibilities are reduced in that group.

Giovanni Andrea Cornia, editor, with Jolly and Stewart, of a UNICEF publication entitled 'Adjustment with a Human Face' says in the first paragraph of the first chapter [10]: 'After almost three decades of steady progress, well-being of children has experienced a marked deterioration in developing countries during the first half of the eighties. Studies made in ten countries show that the nutritional status of children worsens in all of them, with the exception of Korea and Zimbabwe.' Three South American countries, Brazil, Chile and Peru, are among the other eight, as is Jamaica, a Caribbean country.

Talking about this topic at the 9th Latin American Nutrition Congress, held in Puerto Rico last September, I said [11]: 'Ten years ago, in 1979, it was not easy to imagine that, in the upcoming decade, important changes would seriously affect the apparently unstoppable growing process of Latin American countries, several of which were already on the road to development.'

If we take into account that urbanization has been a common phenomenon in the region and that people who moved from rural areas are now unable to cultivate their food because of the limitations of urban life, it follows that nutrition in this context depends largely on the availability of money to buy food at increasing prices, due to the adjustment policies. It is therefore easy to understand that, in this case, motivation about the importance of nutrition and fitness is not enough.

The growing wave of interest in nutrition and fitness has found a big obstacle on its way. People living in cities, motivated day by day about the importance of nutrition and fitness, and willing to do something about it, are now under the impact of economic programs and policies they hardly understand but that nevertheless neutralize such motivation and limit access to the required food that is a fundamental component of the binomial 'nutrition and fitness'.

The problem now is not only the absence of policies; it is also the lack of food and the emotional and physical conditions to exercise.

On the other hand, in those sectors of the population less affected by the adjustment policies in Central and South America, great enthusiasm for walking, jogging, biking, exercising in a fitness center or practicing any sport, while trying to eat in a proper way still exists.

This creates an ideal environment for the interesting programs that are being carried out in different countries. Unfortunately, most of them are still isolated efforts that need to be assembled somehow as coordinated programs. These must be a part of national policies regarding nutrition and physical fitness.

Most of us who work in universities or research institutions believe that education is one of the key tools in the process of enrolling people in the movement to promote health through nutrition and exercise. The same concept can be observed in WHO documents, which state [6]: 'Today, there is a greater need to be aware of how diet and nutrition function and to consciously encourage those eating habits that can help to produce excellence in sports and general well-being.'

In our everyday work, we see how most people are trying to eat well and exercise or practice any sport in an environment full of misconceptions about the role of macro- and micronutrients, and about the truth regarding the best type of exercise, the right time to practice it or the proper clothing to wear.

Sad to say, when they seek the advice of a health professional, most of the time the latter is not fully aware of all the facts or conditions under which the given information can be accepted as valid or applicable. Thus, most of what is now being done in our region tends to solve this problem.

From Country to Country

Most of what is being done in our region is still unpublished information. In order to get a general picture of those isolated efforts I have been talking about, I made a survey covering all Central and South American countries. The information is presented alphabetically by country.

I will begin with the experience of the Clinical Department of the School of Medicine in Botucatu, Brazil. Professors of that Department are carrying out investigations on nutrition and exercise. Evaluation of the nutritional status and metabolic changes and adaptation to different types of physical activities are among their areas of interest. The participation of medical students in their investigations related to nutrition and fitness aims at teaching the new generations of physicians about the role they are expected to play in motivating more people to practice exercise or sports, and to guide them into doing it according to the technical principles universally accepted. Medical students also participate in outpatient clinics dealing with people interested in nutrition and physical fitness [12, 13; Burini, personal commun.].

The Center of Study for Physical Fitness-Research Laboratory, in the same country deserves special reference. They have been working in several areas. In 1987, they defined the physical fitness parameters for the Brazilian population of 7–18 years of age, based on anthropometric, biochemical and maturational data; a unique experience in the region. Differences according to socioeconomical status have also been studied. This year they published an interesting paper analyzing the conditions and problems of sports research in Latin America, presenting realistic and applicable suggestions that I consider to be of great importance for many countries [14, 15; Matsudo, personal commun.].

In Chile, a group from the Department of Food Sciences and Technology is working in the development of nutritional products for athletes according to their specific nutritional requirements, using locally available food sources and technology. Hypercaloric candybars, and others with high protein contents have been in use with good results regarding usefulness and acceptance in their geographical conditions. Isotonic beverages have also been developed [Wittig de Pena, personal commun.].

In Colombia, some schools of dietetics have included in their curricula courses on nutrition and fitness, with varying academic loads. Students participate in various ways; in the evaluation of the nutritional status of athletes and the design and supervision of menus in the cafeterias where they have their meals [Aristizabal, personal commun.].

Later, as professionals, they can participate more fully in programs such as those of Coldeportes, the federal agency for sports, which is working in a research project directed at the morphological, functional and locomotive profile of the Colombian students in order to acquire valuable information to serve as guidelines for action in related areas. They created a foundation to help elite athletes lacking economical support for their careers, also providing them medical, nutritional, social and psychological assistance. Similar nutrition products are being developed in Chile [Noguera, personal commun.].

In the Dominican Republic, a group from the Reid Cabral Hospital in Santo Domingo is planning to offer advice on nutrition and fitness to interested sectors of the population. The subject is also taught in several graduate courses addressed to general practitioners and specialists [Sone, personal commun.].

Guatemala has two important institutions devoted to research in nutrition and related topics. Both of them, the Nutrition Institute of Central America and Panama (INCAP) and the Center for Studies of Senescence and Metabolic Abnormalities (CESSIAM) have researchers interested in nutrition and fitness.

At INCAP, investigations are associated with teaching, as in Brazil, but at a graduate level, more specifically as a part of the Masters on Food and Nutrition program. Among other topics, research projects deal with energy expenditure and physical activities in children and adults, activity patterns related to energy intake and time devoted to usual activities according to such intake. They have also studied physical fitness in relation to type of work in rural and urban populations. The role of anemia in reducing physical performance has also been investigated [16–19; Torun, personal commun.].

The investigations at CESSIAM also include different age groups, vitamin A being one of their main areas of interest. Teaching of this topic is included in courses on Biomedicine and Epidemiology. They also issue a bulletin called 'Avances en Superviviencia Infantil' (Advances in child survival), in which nutrition and physical activities are discussed [Lopez, personal commun.].

The National Institute of Nutrition in Mexico, through its Division of Community Nutrition, participates in activities addressed to athletes with students of different health disciplines such as medicine, nursing and nutrition. Graduate students in their Masters in Public Health program also participate [Martinez, personal commun.].

In Peru, the Department of Nutrition of the German-Peruvian Agreement for Andean Cultures (COPACA) is carrying out studies in the field of nutrition and physical fitness, in relation to work performance in the geographical conditions of the areas where the program is being developed [Maussner, personal commun.].

In Venezuela, the larger universities have integrated nutrition and physical fitness into the curricula of different health studies. This is the case for medicine and dietetics, both at undergraduate and at graduate levels. Research is in progress in the above university schools as well as in private and public institutions interested in sports, noncompetitive physical activities, and in the use of exercise to prevent chronic diseases and for rehabilitation after trauma and cardiological problems.

In spite of the fact that no national policy exists, several activities are carried out on a regular basis, although there is no coordination among them. Nutrition assistance is offered in some sports centers, both through the medical department and through the food services. Two or three times a year, experts from different institutions get together in short courses open to a diverse audience. The general public, athletes, coaches, university students, dietitians and medical personnel have shown a great interest in this topic.

Nutrition and fitness are usually incorporated in the programs at regular meetings, congresses and symposia called by the different professional societies and associations.

I believe that most of the activities that I have mentioned in regard to Venezuela are similarly performed in many other Central and South American countries although the people I interviewed did not mention it, perhaps because of their underestimation of the importance of such low-scale programs.

Conclusion

One of the characteristics of developing countries has been the lack of policies in every field, including that of nutrition and physical fitness. Besides such a fact, most of the programs in this area only consider activities related to competition (sports), leaving aside the growing concern of large sectors of the population for fitness through other types of exercise.

In addition, important negative changes have occurred in the region in the last decade, due to the adjustment policies related to the external debts of all countries. This has determined that after a long-held view of Latin American developing countries as a group of nations moving progressively toward development, they are now in a sharp decline with the majority of their population getting poorer and suffering from a markedly lower household availability of food.

This situation limits the possibility for many people to benefit from the association of nutrition and exercise, in spite of the fact that its importance has been a widely accepted concept in the region.

Although all Central and South American countries share similarities in this regard, the situation differs among them depending on the distribution of people in rural and urban areas. In the countries in which most of the population is still engaged in the traditional hard rural work, lack of exercise is not a problem; however, food shortage and poor sanitation, when present, limit the benefits of such an active life.

In countries with large urban populations, lower household food availability and progressive deterioration of sanitation, and the low levels of physical activity characteristic of urban life, create an inconvenient situation regarding the role of nutrition and fitness as a way to prevent diseases and to enjoy a better quality of life.

For those without such limitations, an important problem is the lack of education programs that should be oriented, both to train professionals dealing with people interested in nutrition and fitness, and to interpret and transmit to the general public the true facts on how nutrition and exercise contribute to fitness.

According to every country's reality in this last decade of the 20th century, efforts should be made to coordinate the ongoing work of isolated groups and to define national policies on nutrition and physical fitness. The socioeconomic situation of Central and South America has changed for the worse, increasing the need for such policies.

References

1 Lara-Pantin E: Policies and programs in nutrition and fitness in Venezuela. Am J Clin Nutr 1989;49:1057–1059.
2 Thairu K: Fitness and nutrition policy in developing nations: Kenya's example. Am J Clin Nutr 1989;49:1054–1056.

3 Horwitz A: Salud, nutricion y desarrollo; in Nutricion un Desafio Nacional. Caracas, Ediciones Fundacion Cavendes, 1985, pp 15–23.
4 Flores R, Immink MDC, Torun B, et al: Functional consequences of marginal malnutrition among agricultural workers in Guatemala. I. Physical Work Capacity. Food Nutr Bull 1984;6:5–11.
5 Streeten P: Lo primero es lo primero. Satisfacer las necesidades humanas basicas en los paises en desarrollo. Madrid, Editorial Tecnos SA, 1986, pp 21–51.
6 Stroot P: A priority for the World Health Organization: Promoting healthy ways of life. Am J Clin Nutr 1989;49:1063–1064.
7 Lara-Pantin E: Obesity in developing countries; in Berry EM, Blondheim SH, Eliahou HE, et al (eds): Recent Advances in Obesity Research. Part V. London, Libbey, 1987, pp 5–8.
8 Roddick J: The dance of millions: Latin America and the debt crisis. London, Latin America Bureau (Research Action) Ltd, 1988, pp 4–17.
9 Fundacredesa: 15 años investigando para el mejor conocimiento de Venezuela. Caracas, Ediciones de la Presidencia de la Republica de Venezuela, 1991, p 30.
10 Cornia GA: Declive economico y bienestar humano en la primera mitad de los años ochenta; in Cornia GA, Jolly Y, Stewart F (eds): Ajuste con Rostro Humano. Proteccion de los Grupos Vulnerables y Promocion del Crecimiento. Madrid, Siglo XX de España Editores SA, 1987, vol I, pp 14–40.
11 Lara-Pantin E: Iberoamerica, un paso atras forzado por la crisis. Arch Latinoam Nutr 1992;42;in press.
12 Anselmo MAC, Mathias MRC, Gaiotto ME, Cervi EC, Burini RC: Avaliacao do estado nutricional de jovens atletas nadadores e corredores (fundistas). XII Jornada Científica de Botucatu (SP), Anais, p 119.
13 Cervi EC, Matsubara BB, Mathias MRC, Curi PR, Burini RC: Plasma energy-yielding substrates and cardiovascular parameters changes during exhaustive-treadmill exercise and relationship to training levels in healthy young subjects. Sci Mov 1989;3:17–25.
14 Matsudo VH: Motor fitness characteristics of Brazilian boys and girls from 7 to 18 years of age. Sport Sci Rev 1987;10:55–61.
15 Matsudo VR: Present conditions and problems of sports research in Latin America from the point of view of international cooperation. Sci Mov 1992;6:63–74.
16 Torun B: Physiological measurements of physical activities among children under free-living conditions; in Pollit E, Amante P (eds): Energy Intake and Activity. New York, Liss, 1984, pp 159–184.
17 Torun B: Energy cost of various physical activities in healthy children; in Sturch B, Scrimshaw N (eds): Activity, Energy Expenditure and Energy Requirements of Infants and Children. Lausanne, IDECG, 1990, pp 139–183.
18 Torun B: Incremento de la actividad fisica mediante mejoria del estado nutricional. Arch Latinoam Nutr 1989;39:308–326.
19 Vitery FE, Torun B: Anaemia and physical work capacity. Clin Haematol 1974;3: 609–626.

Eleazar Lara-Pantin, Unidad de Investigaciones en Nutricion, Apartado 3458, Valencia 2002 A (Venezuela)

Simopoulos AP (ed): Nutrition and Fitness in Health and Disease.
World Rev Nutr Diet. Basel, Karger, 1993, vol 72, pp 200–205

Trends in Physical Fitness and Nutrition in the USA

York Onnen

Director of Program Development, President's Council on Physical Fitness and Sports, Washington, D.C., USA

Introduction

The paper presented by the President's Council on Physical Fitness and Sports (PCPFS) at the First International Conference on Nutrition and Fitness in 1988, under the patronage of the IOC and the WHO, outlined the organizational structure and programs of the United States government in partnership with private industry.

What is important to understand when one examines the trends and projections of physical fitness, sports and their relationship to nutrition as experienced in the USA, is that there is no single agency or organization in government or the private sector with overall responsibility for these areas.

Consequently, it is difficult at best to receive an accurate and comprehensive overview of what nearly 249 million Americans are doing to exercise and eat right at any given time.

Status of Youth Fitness and Health

One agency that has played a significant role in the development of policies and directions that many international visitors see as an essential checkpoint is the President's Council on Physical Fitness and Sports (PCPFS).

Established in 1956 as the President's Council on Youth Fitness in response to a study conducted by Hans Kraus, MD, and his colleagues Bonnie Prudden and Sonja Weber who found American youngsters of that era came up short when compared with their European counterparts using a few simple fitness tests, the PCPFS' predecessor established a network of public and private organizations who would take steps to remedy the shortcomings.

Subsequently, major national advertising campaigns featuring films, television and radio messages, as well as magazine and newspaper advertisements and articles fueled a national awakening. Schools created high-energy physical education programs. Sports at all levels became a way of life for millions of youth. Every community placed high priorities on hiring qualified teachers and leaders.

For many of us who grew up in the 1950s and 1960s, the problem appeared to be fixed. Other priorities began to take the place of physical education in the schools. And another generation began to emerge in the 1970s and 1980s, one that had not been exposed to the awakening of the Eisenhower-Kennedy years.

At the same time, a growing concern over the health of the population and the rapidly growing cost of health care, refocused public attention away from what many felt was a job accomplished.

As a consequence, today's youth are once again at risk. Not a single one of the 50 states offers daily physical education from kindergarten through the twelfth grade (the report to the 1988 conference mentioned Illinois as the only state with a K-12 daily requirement but only two-thirds of the schools actually fulfill the mandate).

Other reports such as the Chrysler/AAU Study, the Health-Related Youth Fitness Survey and the School Population Youth Fitness Survey confirmed that America's youth of the 1980s and 1990s had not improved their fitness or health compared to the earlier generation but in many cases were turning into the proverbial couch potatoes. The apparent causes? Too much TV, not enough physical activity. More automobiles and less walking. Massive cutbacks in physical education in the schools and a growing reliance on home, work and leisure conveniences.

Once again, America's youth are at risk. Nearly 40% of those between the ages of 5 and 8 exhibit a major risk factor for heart disease and youth of all ages today are significantly fatter than their counterparts in 1975.

The past decade has seen the introduction of major new initiatives in the USA that promise to put the nation's youth back on track. *Healthy*

People 2000 is one of those initiatives which has received input from hundreds of public and private institutions responding to the US Public Health Service's lead.

Others include the Fit to Achieve program of the National Association of Sport and Physical Education (NASPE), the Fun and Fitness Program of the National Recreation and Park Association (NRPA), the national fitness and sports programs such as Hershey's Track and Field Program, the Marine Corps Youth Fitness Program and the National Guard Bureau's Youth Fitness Program.

Another major initiative undertaken by PCPFS Chairman Arnold Schwarzenegger was to visit all 50 states, meet with each governor and conduct a summit within each state bringing together those organizations and leaders who worked with the nation's youth.

While it took nearly three and a half years to complete the tours – the final state visit was accomplished in April 1992 – substantive changes to how states perceived the problem of youth fitness and began to implement measurable strategies became apparent almost immediately, largely through the tremendous popularity of the former President's representative, Arnold Schwarzenegger, and the alliance of such powerful groups as the American Alliance on Health, Physical Education, Recreation and Dance (AAHPERD), the National Association of Governor's Councils and Physical Fitness and Sports (NAGCPF&S) and the PCPFS.

A conference sponsored by the Sporting Goods Manufacturers Association and conducted in Washington, D.C. in 1991, the National Youth Fitness Summit, brought together dozens of organizations that are now working together to improve the fitness *and* health status of America's youth.

Middle-Aged Adults and the Fitness Revolution

Middle-aged men and women in America became the soldiers in the Fitness Revolution that took place during the 1970s and 1980s – fueled by a new focus on aerobics, the brainchild of Dr. Kenneth Cooper – where cardiorespiratory and cardiovascular fitness became the rage. Millions took up running and the milder version, jogging.

During this time, sporting goods manufacturing developed into a thirty-billion dollar annual industry and Americans in every walk of life sought to improve their exercise habits *and* the way they ate.

The PCPFS, along with its partners in the public and private sectors, began to espouse the essential relationship between physical activity and nutrition which today is the subject of this second international conference. Major public health initiatives such as the National High Blood Pressure Education Program, the National Cholesterol Education Program, the National Osteoporosis Prevention campaign and others focusing on similar risk factors incorporated the exercise and nutrition message.

May Becomes a Time of Renewed Life

Beginning in 1983, the PCPFS launched the month of May as National Physical Fitness and Sports Month, to enable communities across the land to join in a celebration of sports for all. The campaign recognized the involvement of many segments of society that already observed the month, most notably older Americans, the high blood pressure community and lifetime sports such as bicycling and tennis.

To assure that the nation's physical educators and sports devotees were recognized, the first week in May became National Physical Education and Sport Week.

Today, the month is introduced to the nation through the Great American Workout held on May 1; the past 3 years have brought sports, government and movie celebrities to the White House South Lawn for an early-morning, nationally televised exercise demonstration which featured President and Mrs. Bush, PCPFS Chairman Arnold Schwarzenegger, Cabinet members and other prominent exercisers.

Older Americans Become Top Priority

At the beginning of the 20th century, less than 1 in 10 Americans was age 55+ and only 1 in 25 was age 65+. Today, 1 in 5 is at least 55 years old and 1 in 8 is at least 65.

The projected growth in the older population is expected to raise the median age of the US population to 36 by the year 2000, to 42 by the year 2030, and to 43 by the year 2040.

Life expectancy for both men and women continues to rise although the rate of increase has slowed somewhat and major segments of the population such as blacks and Hispanics are less fortunate.

Older Americans are at a critical point in terms of the nation's health care system and their ability to pay for life's essentials. More and more of the nation's priorities call for prevention of diseases and chronic illnesses to forestall the seemingly inevitable high cost of growing older.

The nation's effort is now directed toward re-introducing physical activity as an essential element of successful aging.

At the turn of the century, most of the population lived and worked on the farm in a rural setting. Life was physically demanding for city dwellers as well.

Today, just 2% of the population lives on the farm and even there automation has removed much of the physical demand.

Recent surveys conducted by the US National Center for Health Statistics (NCHS) suggest that only 8% of the older population exercises at a sufficient level and duration to promote heart health. Furthermore, most older adults are ignorant about the type of physical activity that is appropriate to them to promote safety and prevent chronic illnesses.

In addition, survey results from the US Centers for Disease Control (CDC) report that little change has occurred in the exercise habits of most Americans, including older adults, in the past 10 years.

The PCPFS has embarked on a path to get more adults to exercise properly and to incorporate the message on the importance of nutrition as an element of that message.

Public and private sector initiatives will be engaged to turn around the fitness habits of all Americans. Through activities such as the President's Challenge, the Presidential Sports Award and Senior Games youth and older adults alike will be encouraged to exercise and eat right, to assure that America enters the 21st century a healthier, fitter nation.

Conclusion

Americans face a dilemma in that society's increasing dependence on technology in daily living – mass transportation, television, home and work automated systems and a myriad of other conveniences – have greatly reduced the amount of physical activity that the human body needs for health and well-being.

Although research indicates that at present the population of the United States on average lives longer and enjoys a high quality of life with greater sports and leisure time participation than in the past, many Americans do not avail themselves of physical activity throughout life.

The Nation's schools continue to place a low priority on physical education with only 1 of 50 states mandating physical education from kindergarten through the 12th grade. For older adults, the majority of the population does not understand or practice physical activity that clearly relates to health and safety risk factors such as heart disease, chronic low back pain and a variety of other life-style-related illnesses.

The President's Council on Physical Fitness and Sports believes in the essential nature of daily exercise and the important relationship between physical activity and nutrition. It is the lead Federal agency in the Nation's plan to improve public health under Healthy People 2000. Serving as a catalyst and presidential advisory body, the Council has set ambitious goals to improve the health and well-being of Americans of every age, gender, race and religion.

York E. Onnen, Director of Program Development, President's Council on Physical Fitness and Sports, Suite 250, 701 Pennsylvania Avenue, N.W., Washington, DC 20004 (USA)

Simopoulos AP (ed): Nutrition and Fitness in Health and Disease.
World Rev Nutr Diet. Basel, Karger, 1993, vol 72, pp 206–217

Policies and Programs in Nutrition and Physical Fitness in Greece[1]

Anthony Kafatos, George Mamalakis

University of Crete, School of Medicine,
Department of Social and Preventive Medicine, Iraklion, Crete, Greece

Introduction

There is abundant archaeological evidence indicating that the ancient Greeks were among the first, if not the first, to realize the interdependence of mind and body. According to an ancient Greek saying, 'a healthy mind resides in a healthy body and vice versa'. The ancient Greeks were probably the first to understand the significance of both diet and exercise in the maintenance of a healthy body and spirit. The emphasis placed upon exercise and proper diet becomes evident by Hippocrates' writings and in that the Olympic games originated in ancient Greece. The diet of ancient Greeks was simple and consisted of bread, olive oil, pulses, fruit, vegetable, fish and milk products. Meat was rarely consumed, primarily on special occasions and festivities. As a result of this diet and life-style, modern Greeks were found to have the lowest coronary heart disease mortality among other developed countries.

In the early 1960s, mortality statistics indicated that the death rate of Greeks due to arteriosclerotic and degenerative heart disease was seven times lower than that of American men of the same age [1]. Similar observations were made in 1978 [3] when Cretan farmers were compared with their American counterparts [2]. Data from the 1960s and the 1970s indicated that Crete and Corfu, two of the islands of Greece, had the lowest mortality due to coronary artery disease compared to 7 other countries [3–5]. Up until recently, Crete had been associated with low mortality rates

[1] Supported by the European Economic Community through the integrated Mediterranean program of Crete and the Greek Ministry of Health.

for ischaemic heart disease [4, 3, 6–9, 10], a fact that had been attributed primarily to the dietary habits of Cretans [3, 4].

There are archaeological data indicating that at least up until the mid 1950s Cretans had been maintaining dietary habits similar to those during the Minoan age (1200 BC) [11]. The traditional Cretan diet included wheat-based products, legumes, an abundance of home-grown vegetables, seasonal fruit, milk and milk products. The consumption of meat and fish was limited and the major source of calories was provided by home-baked whole-wheat bread, olives, and olive oil. Forty percent of the calories were derived from fat and most of it, approximately 33%, was derived from monounsaturated fat, oleic acid in particular, 12% from protein, and the rest from complex carbohydrates. Perhaps the most unique feature of the traditional Cretan diet was, however, the use of olive oil as a major source of calories. The biochemical role of such increased amounts of oleic acid in the atherogenic process is not yet known. Nevertheless, among other factors (e.g. low intake of saturated fat, slow pace of life, relatively competition-free culturally sanctioned modes of acting, type B behavior), this extensive use of olive oil has been suspected as a main reason for the low incidence of myocardial infarction in Crete [3, 4].

Cardiovascular Risk Factors, Diet and Physical Activity in Middle-Aged and Elderly Greeks

Relatively recent data have indicated shifts in both diet and physical fitness of Greeks. A cross-sectional study of Cretan fathers and their children indicated that there had been a 25% increase in serum cholesterol in Cretan fathers between the mid-1960s and the late 1970s [3, 9]. The particular increase reflected a corresponding shift in the dietary habits of Cretans that was confirmed also through serum lipid and adipose tissue fatty acid analyses [12]. Also, a recent study of a representative sample of middle-class Cretans showed that over the last 26 years there has been a rise in serum cholesterol concentration by 36% (fig. 1) and a consumption of a diet that although still high in fat, has changed to include increased amounts of meat and cheese (saturated fat) and in which the consumption of monounsaturated fat has decreased [13] (tables 1, 2). There has also been a decrease in physical activity. Most of the subjects (70%) could be classified as sedentary, 20% walked 2–4 km/day and only a minority (10%) engaged daily in some kind of physical activity (fig. 2). The particular

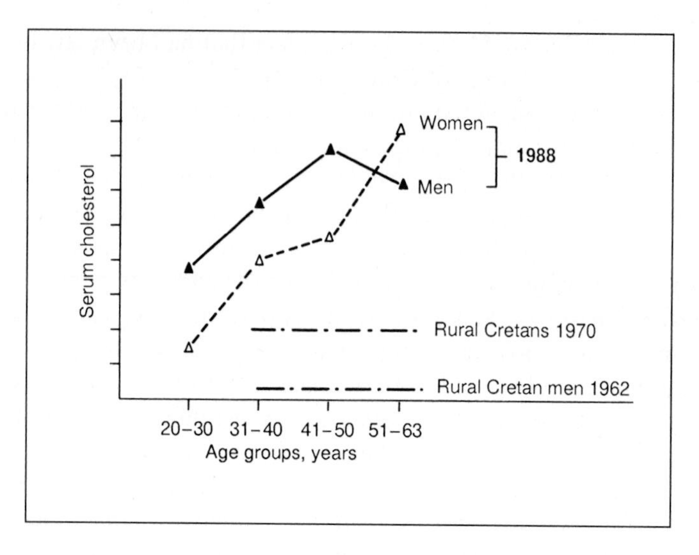

Fig. 1. Mean total serum cholesterol in Cretan men and women.

Table 1. Food consumption patterns in Cretan men

Food Items	1960 (n = 31) g/day	1988 (n = 182) g/day	p one-sample t test
Bread	380	114.78 ± 79.78	<0.001
Cereals	30	29.09 ± 81.23	
Potatoes	190	88.35 ± 130.83	<0.001
Pulses	30	40.52 ± 108.16	
Vegetables	191	238.34 ± 196.31	<0.01
Fruit	464	322.31 ± 313.17	<0.001
Meat	35	91.20 ± 117.76	<0.001
Fish	18	34.04 ± 73.69	<0.01
Eggs	25	13.08 ± 44.45	<0.01
Cheese	13	60.58 ± 75.89	<0.001
Milk	235	57.84 ± 116.68	<0.001
Edible fats	95	49.96 ± 39.64	<0.001
Sugar products	20	20.59 ± 21.45	
Pastries	–	64.59 ± 169.35	
Alcohol, 100%	15	10.15 ± 19.86	<0.01
Rest	107	161.61 ± 221.88	<0.001

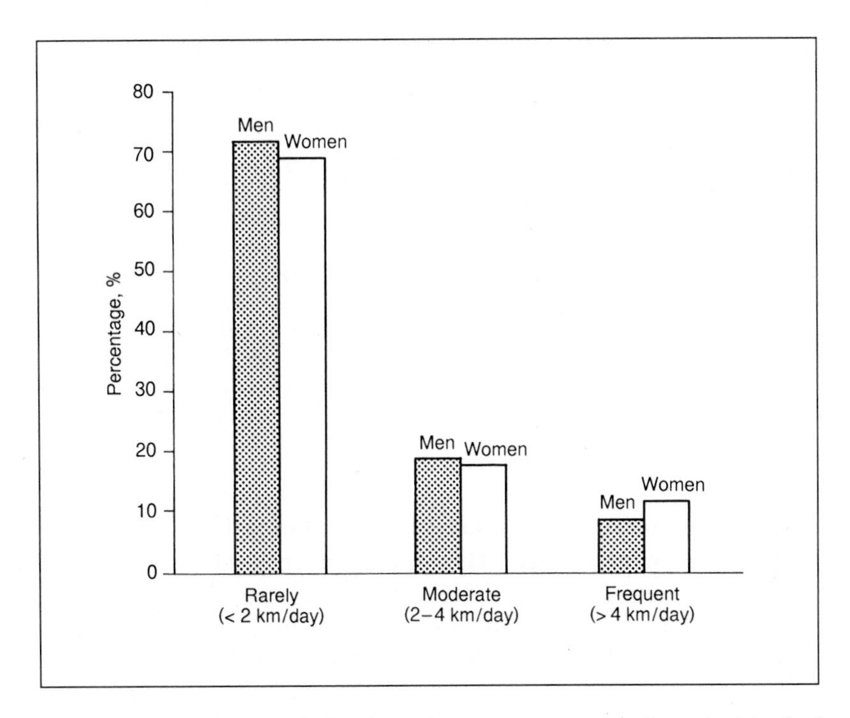

Fig. 2. Daily walking by middle class urban men and women from the island of Crete.

Table 2. Dietary energy derived from fat

Variable	Cretan men 1960 (ages 40–59)	Men 1988 (ages 40–60) (n = 181)	Women 1988 (n = 131)
Total fat	123	98.9±47.5	89.97±46.96
Total fat, % energy	40	35.8	41.75
Saturated fatty acids, % energy	8	10.20	13.4
Monounsaturated fatty acids, % energy	29	17.0	18.29
Polyunsaturated fatty acids, % energy	3	3	3.55
Cholesterol intake, mg/1,000 kcal	125	110	108
P:S	0.37	0.28	0.26
M:S	3.62	1.66	1.37

Table 3. Risk factor status of Cretan men and women [13]

Risk factors[1]	Men, %	Women, %
0	3.8	20.6
1	18.3	42
2	41.3	27.5
>3	36.6	9.9

[1] BMI > 26 kg/m^2; smoking > 10 cigarettes/day; serum cholesterol > 5.2 mmol/l; systolic BP > 140 mm Hg; diastolic BP > 90; medical history of CHD and family history of CHD.

observations are in sharp contrast to those during 1960, when most subjects walked on the average 10 km/day and/or engaged regularly in physical labor. The dietary changes observed in other populations, such as for example the Dutch in the Zutphen study, during approximately the same time period (1962–1985), are quite different [14]. Although the mean serum cholesterol levels are approximately the same today in Dutch and Cretan middle-aged men, the coronary heart disease (CHD) mortality rates have been decreasing in the Dutch (–11% men) and increasing in Greeks (+14%) during the last 30-year period [15]. The incidence of coronary heart disease risk factors in middle-aged Greeks is presented in table 3 [13].

In 1991 the Department of Social Medicine, University of Crete, conducted a follow-up study of those men who had participated in the Seven Countries study in 1960 [4]. From the surviving 336 men (668 in 1960), 293 consented to be examined. Of those 293 men, 85 were then randomly selected and dietary data were obtained (quantitative frequency of food consumption). Fifty-seven of those 85 men were in the 70- to 91-year age group. Out of those 57 men, a random sample of 21 people was then selected and weighted food intakes were taken on 3 consecutive days. The results of the weighted food intake appear in table 4. The monounsaturated fat intake significantly decreased from 29% in 1960 to 23.3% in 1991 ($p < 0.005$), while the saturated fat intake increased from 8 to 9.6% ($p < 0.005$). Dietary cholesterol decreased from 100 to 150 mg/1,000 kcal in 1960 to 84 mg/1,000 kcal in 1991 ($p < 0.005$), probably due to the decrease in the consumption of eggs. It appears that overall there had been

Table 4. Food-consumption patterns in Cretan men

Food items	1960 (n = 31) g/day	1991 (n = 21) g/day	% change
Cereals	30*	161*	436
Pulses	30*	93*	210
Vegetables	191*	336*	76
Meat	35	46	31
Fish	18**	58**	222
Cheese	13	24	85
Milk	235	228	-3
Alcohol	15	13	-13
Bread	380*	187*	-51
Potatoes	190*	78*	-59
Fruit	464*	232*	-50
Eggs	25*	10*	-60
Sugar products	20	17	-15

t tests; * $p < 0.005$; ** $p < 0.01$.

a deterioration in the dietary habits of the particular sample over the 30-year period between 1960 and 1991. Follow-ups of the 40- to 59-year old cohort of men who had initially participated in the seven-countries study indicated that there had been a 15% increase in total serum cholesterol (TSC) from 1960 to 1970 and a subsequent minor decrease in 1991. Overall, there had been an 11% increase of TSC during the last 31 years [unpubl. data]. Similar increases have been observed in body mass index and in systolic and diastolic blood pressures (table 5).

During the last 30 years Greece has been going through rapid technological and socioeconomic change. The annual per capita income has increased from $ 300 in 1960 to $ 6,536 in 1990 (363% increase excluding an approximate 20% annual inflation rate during this period of 30 years). Life has grown faster and there are fast-food stores even in the rural areas. Over the last 30 years the typical Cretan has become more prosperous and has switched from farming to business, primarily tourism. Most importantly, his dietary habits are being westernized. There has been a shift towards materialism, over-achievement (getting to the top) and competi-

Table 5. Total serum cholesterol, anthropometric and blood pressure measurements in the Cretan cohort of men 40–59 years of age in 1960 from the seven-countries study who survived in 1991 [unpubl. data]

Dates of follow-up	n	1960		1965		1970		1991	
		$\overline{X}$	SD	$\overline{X}$	SD	$\overline{X}$	SD	$\overline{X}$	SD
Total serum cholesterol, mmol/l	198	5.2*	1	5.6*	1	6*	1	5.8*	1.1
Weight, kg	228	64*	9.3	65.8*	9.9	67.6*	10.7	68.7*	13.1
Height, cm	225	166.5*	5.9	166*	6.5	166.4*	6.2	164.2*	6.6
BMI, kg/m^2	225	23.1*	3	23.8*	3.1	24.4*	3.4	25.5*	4.7
Systolic BP, mm Hg	181	133.6*	16.9	129.1*	18.1	130.5*	20.2	162.4*	23.0
Diastolic BP 5th phase, mm Hg	181	80*	11.3	78.8*	12	76.5*	10.8	89.1*	10.1

Analysis of variance: * $p < 0.001$.

tive interpersonal situations. Also, life has become more sedentary, in our opinion partly due to the fact that television has entered almost all Greek households. This particular phenomenon may impose a greater threat on younger generations. The urban population of Greece has increased over the last 30 years because of a trend from a large part of the rural population towards migrating to urban centers such as Athens. Greece is now considered to be among the developed countries, and has begun to manifest the epidemiological characteristics of western societies.

Cardiovascular Risk Factors in Greek Children

Table 6 reviews the total serum cholesterol levels in Greek children for the last 23 years. There is a definite trend towards higher total serum cholesterol levels in children from 1969 to 1992. Although the comparisons are difficult because of difference in age, sex, phase of adolescent growth and place of residence, overall it appears that the levels of serum cholesterol in children have increased. Again, as with the adults, the chief reason for the particular increase is the socioeconomic changes that have been occurring in Greece during the last decades. As shown in table 6,

Table 6. Total serum cholesterol in Greek children

Study	Years of study							
	1969	1973	1977	1979	1980	1985	1987	1992
Rural Greece [28] (boys under 6–12 years)	3.5							
Rural central Greece [29]		4.3						
Athens		5.4						
Crete urban + rural [12]								
5–9%			4.5					
10–14%			4.8					
Athenian children (10–14 years), plasma cholesterol, 113 boys and girls [17]				3.9				
Thrace (5 years) [30]								
Boys				3.4				
Girls				3.6				
Crete (5 years; urban + rural)								
Boys				3.2				
Girls				3.4				
Cross-cultural study [31], (boys 9–17 years)								
Iraklion								
9 years old					4.2			
12 years old					4.0			
15 years old					4.4			
Athens								
9 years old					4.6			
12 years old					4.3			
15 years old					4.1			
Rural Crete [32]								
Timbaki 5–9 years						4.0		
10–14 years						4.4		
15–18 years						4.0		
Anogia 5–9 years						4.1		
10–14 years						3.7		
15–18 years						3.8		
Rural Crete (seven countries area) [22]						4.4		
Rural Crete [27]								
St Vassilios (12–14 years, girls)							4.4	
Amari (12–14 years, girls)							3.9	
Urban Crete								
St Nicholas [unpubl.]								
Boys (13 years old)								4.7
Girls (13 years old)								4.9

children from Saint Vassilios village, a tourism center, have higher serum cholesterol levels (4.4 mmol/l) than children from Amari (3.9 mmol/l), a non-touristic area maintaining to a larger degree the traditional Cretan way of life. Much larger differences can be seen between Saint Nicholas town, one of the most highly developed touristic areas, and Amari and Anogia, two non-touristic areas. The population sample employed consisted of 13-year-old boys and girls and the TSC levels observed were 4.8 mmol/l for Saint Nicholas, 3.9 mmol/l for Amari, and 3.7 mmol/l for Anogia. The laboratory determinations in these three areas were performed by the Department of Social Medicine participation in an external quality control program. A cross-cultural study involving 139 boys aged 8–16 years indicated statistically significant differences in the adipose tissue monounsaturated fat between those living in Athens, a large metropolitan city, and those living in Iraklion, a smaller city in Crete. The Athens cohort had significantly lower levels of monounsaturated fat than that of Iraklion city, and the particular phenomenon is thought of as resulting from the adoption of a dietary pattern more similar to that of western societies from the part of those inhabiting large metropolitan areas of Greece [16]. A similar study involving 1,113 ten- to 15-year-old boys and girls that attended public schools in the area of Athens indicated that over one third (34%) of the particular population had one or more risk factors (hypertension, hypercholesterolemia, smoking and obesity, weight above the 90th percentile) for cardiovascular disease [17]. The high prevalence of obesity among the particular adolescents is in accord with data from the Greek island of Crete where 31% of the infants aged 12–15 months have a relative weight greater than 110% [18, 19]. The explanation for the particular phenomenon lies in the poor health and nutrition knowledge of Greek parents coupled with a tendency to overfeed their children and the limited physical activity permitted in large and densely populated cities like Athens. Other studies have also pointed out a high incidence of obesity [20] and smoking [21] among Greek children. A relatively recent study in 1987 indicated that 97 Cretan boys 7–9 years of age had significantly higher serum total cholesterol levels than their American counterparts [22]. The particular observations are alarming in light of the evidence that possible risk factors for CHD at an early age persist into adulthood [23–25] or that the major risk factors leading to CHD have their roots in childhood [26]. The high prevalence of cardiovascular risk factors in younger generations of Greeks is thus expected to increase morbidity and mortality from cardiovascular diseases and requires appropriate preventive measures.

Table 7. Mean serum cholesterol and LDL at baseline and adjusted changes in the intervention and control groups after 1 year of intervention [27]

	Intervention group, mg/dl		Control group, mg/dl	
	$\overline{X}$	SD	$\overline{X}$	SD
Total serum cholesterol				
Value at baseline	170.3	-25.8	151	-23.5
Adjusted change	0.7	-27.8	17.9	-22.1
LDL-Cholesterol				
Value at baseline	110.2	-22.6	90.3	-20.1
Adjusted change	0.01	-25.7	17.6	-20.8

Despite the alarming facts already presented, there is no national policy on nutrition, physical fitness and prevention in Greece. Only isolated, scattered and inadequately funded efforts towards prevention have been taking place the last decade. The only physical fitness programs conducted on a national basis are those during primary and secondary education. Physical education, approximately 2–3 h of instruction per week, is part of the curriculum of all primary and secondary schools. However, the particular educational program focuses exclusively on physical fitness (gymnastics and sports), while no emphasis is given on the nutritional component. Physical education classes are conducted by primary school teachers during primary education and by physical education graduates during secondary education. There are currently four Greek Universities with physical education departments. A pilot study conducted by the Department of Social Medicine, University of Crete, in a small number of schools yielded positive results. The particular study, an educational intervention program for the prevention of cardiovascular disease, indicated that the intervention group showed more favorable shifts in total serum cholesterol, diastolic pressure, body mass index, smoking and knowledge of health issues [27] (table 7).

In conclusion, the high saturated fat intake by contemporary Greeks combined with the diminishing monounsaturated fat intake and the low energy expenditure in physical activity leads to high obesity rates and high total serum cholesterol rates as compared to levels three decades ago. As a result the cardiovascular mortality rate is rapidly increasing in Greece during the last decades. It is therefore urgent to establish a national research center for nutrition, physical fitness and preventive medicine. The particular center will coordinate and expand current programs and will advise Greek government on a national policy on nutrition and fitness.

References

1 World Health Organization: Annual Epidemiological and Vital Statistics for 1960. Geneva, WHO, 1963, p 449.
2 Kuller LH: The epidemiology of cardiovascular disease in current perspectives. Am J Epidemiol 1976;104:425.
3 Christakis G, Severinghaus EL, Maldonado Z, et al: Crete: A study in metabolic epidemiology of coronary heart disease. Am J Cardiol 1965;15:320–332.
4 Keys A: Coronary heart disease in seven countries. Circulation 1970;41(suppl 1): 1–211.
5 Aravanis C, Dontas A: 17-year mortality from coronary heart disease in the Greek islands heart study. Abstr 18th Ann Conf Cardiovascular Disease, Epidemiology. Orlando, 1978.
6 Keys A (ed): Seven Countries: A Multivariate Analysis of Death and Coronary Heart Diseases. Cambridge, Harvard University Press 1980.
7 Kafatos AG, Christakis G: Pediatric nutritional determinants of chronic diseases. J Florida Med Assoc 1979;66:436.
8 Kafatos AG, Christakis G, Fordyce M, et al: Coronary heart disease (CHD) risk factors status of children of MI and non-MI fathers in Crete, Greece. Federation Proceedings 1979;Part I Vol 38:446.
9 Kafatos AG, Kenne E, Kafatos E, et al: The dietary intake of Cretan men with premature myocardial infarction (MI) and their children in comparison to two non-MI groups of men and their children. Iatriki 1979;35:268–279.
10 Keys A: Coronary heart disease. The global picture. Atherosclerosis 1978;22:149–192.
11 Allbaugh LG: Crete: A case study of an underdeveloped area. Princeton, Princeton University Press, 1953.
12 Kafatos AG, Nikolaidis G, Kafatos E, et al: Risk factor status of Myocardial Infarction (MI) and non-MI subjects and their children in Crete. Volume of Abstracts. Athens International Symposium on the Child in the World of Tomorrow, Athens, July 2–8, 1978.
13 Kafatos A, Kouroumalis I, Vlachonikolis I, et al: Coronary-heart-disease risk-factor status of the Cretan urban population in the 1980s. Am J Clin Nutr 1991;54:591–598.
14 Kromhout D, Keys A, Aravanis C, et al: Food consumption patterns in the 1960s in seven countries. Am J Clin Nutr 1989;49:889–894.
15 World Health Organization: World Health Statistics Annual 1988. Geneva, World Health Organization, 1988.

16 Fordyce MK, Christakis G, Kafatos G, et al: Adipose tissue fatty acid composition of adolescents in a US-Greece cross-cultural study of coronary heart disease risk factors. J Chron Dis 1983;36:481–486.
17 Kafatos AG, Panagiotakopoulos G, Bastakis N, et al: Cardiovascular risk factor status of Greek adolescents in Athns. Prevent Med 1981;10:173–186.
18 Kafatos AG: Obesity in infancy and childhood. Iatriki 1978;34:290–308.
19 Kafatos aG, Bada A, Pantelakis S, et al: Infant mortality and morbidity in three counties of Greece (relations with medical and socio-cultural factors). Iatriki 1978; 33:39–49.
20 Kafatos AG, Panagiotakopoulos G, Trakas D, et al: The epidemiology of cardiovascular risk factors in Greek children aged 13, in comparison to children from 11 other countries. Iatriki 1981;40:113–121.
21 Kafatos AG, Trakas D, Saraphidou G, et al: Smoking among children aged 10–14 in Athens, Greece. Iatriki 1981;40:373–379.
22 Aravanis C, Mensink RP, Karalias N, et al: Serum lipids, apoproteins and nutrient intake in rural Cretan boys consuming high-olive-oil diets. J Clin Epidemiol 1988; 41:1117–1123.
23 Berenson GS: Cardiovascular Risk Factors in Children. New York, Oxford University Press, 1980.
24 Lauer RM, Shekelle RB: Childhood Prevention of Atherosclerosis and Hypertension. New York, Raven Press, 1980.
25 Williams CL: Pediatric Risk factors for Major Chronic Disease. St Louis, Warren Green, 1984.
26 Kannel WB, Dawber TR: Atherosclerosis as a pediatric problem. J Pediatr 1972;80: 544–554.
27 Lionis C, Kafatos A, Vlachonikolis I, et al: The effects of a health education intervention program among Cretan adolescents. Prevent Med 1991;20:685–699.
28 Mayo O, Frasser GR, Stamatoyannopoulos G: Genetic influences on serum cholesterol in two Greek villages. Hum Hered 1969;19–86.
29 Papadopoulos N, Sakellaropoulos D: Serum cholesterol levels of Greek children. Iatriki 1973;24:396.
30 Kafatos A, Ioannou E, Papaioannou C, et al: Risk factors for cardiovascular diseases in children 5 years old from two areas of Greece with extreme indices of infant mortality. Iatriki 1983;45:221–228.
31 Christakis G, Kafatos A, Fordyce M, et al: Cross-cultural determinants coronary heart disease risk factors in adolescents: A USA-Greece cross-cultural study-preliminary results. Nutrition in Health and Disease and International Development. Symposia from the XII International Congress of Nutrition. New York, Liss, 1981; pp 20–31.
32 Kafatos A, Manesis E: Epidemiology of chronic pesticide exposure in a rural Cretan Community. Iatriki 1989;56:517–575.

Anthony Kafatos, University of Crete, School of Medicine,
Department of Social and Preventive Medicine,
POB 1393, Iraklion, Crete (Greece)

Simopoulos AP (ed): Nutrition and Fitness in Health and Disease.
World Rev Nutr Diet. Basel, Karger, 1993, vol 72, pp 218–226

Nutrition and Body Build: A Kenyan Review[1]

Meke Mukeshi[a], *Kihumbu Thairu*[b]

[a]Department of Medical Physiology, Faculty of Medicine, University of Nairobi, Kenya; [b]Commonwealth Secretariat, Marlborough House, London, UK

Introduction

Four years ago during the first conference on nutrition and fitness, the panel summaries indicated that organized policies and programs on nutrition and fitness were nonexistent in developing countries. One of the problems of formulating these is the lack of scientific knowledge necessary for the formulation, especially since other more deserving priorities such as calorie malnutrition are evident in many sectors [1]. This gap in knowledge is crucial as a precedent since it is necessary to guarantee an audience as well as motivate policy makers that there is a need for these programs based on sound scientific principles. In view of the above, since no scientific data was available, we decided to collect relevant data as well as analyze and present ongoing research to authenticate our case.

In the first investigation spanning a period of 4 years, the goal was to test the hypothesis that food intake is causally related to functional consequences. This group (nonathletes) was primarily farm workers. They exhibited low education, low socioeconomic status, and no running water or electricity in the households.

A subsequent investigation was carried out in a high performance group which included highly trained runners. The latter were urbanized pastoralists who should have participated in an international event in 5,000 m or longer at least 3 months prior to testing.

[1] This study was supported by the University of Nairobi and USAID grant No. DAN-1309-G-SS-1070-00.

Although more than 3,000 individuals were investigated, the data analysis and hence presentation has only been done on a proportion due to logistics and costs.

Materials and Methods

All individuals underwent a physical examination. Standardized questionnaires were used to assess income, education status and family history. Lung function, strength tests, resting energy expenditure and maximal oxygen consumption were evaluated in selected individuals. Blood samples were obtained and assessed for hemoglobin (Hb), hematocrit (Hct), serum ferritin as well as the presence of malarial parasites. Stool and urine analysis were also carried out. Food intake was evaluated 2 days per month using a combination of recall and direct observation (also important for validation). Therefore, 3 months were adequate since 6 days are representative of 'usual' intake. The detailed methodologies have been summarized elsewhere [2].

Results

The results of the preliminary analysis were as follows. Table 1 summarizes some of the physical and physiological characteristics. The age range was 19–31 YOA. The average calorie intake for a 1-year analysis in the non-athletic individuals ranged from 1,684 to 2,338 kcal/day for males and 1,382 to 2,015 kcal/day for females. The mean energy and the proportions of the nutrients consumed are depicted in table 2. The proportion of animal proteins consumed is also calculated.

Daily carbohydrate (CHO) intake averaged 75% of total energy whereas protein (PR) and lipids contributed on average 11 and 13.5%, respectively. A comparison of total intakes to reference values indicate apparent lower intakes among Kenyans (table 3).

Figures 1 and 2 summarize the energy intakes, resting metabolic rate (RMR), weight and fatness in males and females, respectively. Energy intake and fatness are in congruence except during the planting season, whereby in females the fatness decreases while body weight increases due to higher levels of physical activity.

The mean RMR was 23.6 and 23.5 kcal/kg for males and females, respectively. During the observation period, there was a drought (July to December) and the intake decreased by 19% (401 kcal) and 23% (433 kcal) in males and females, respectively. However, no difference in RMR was observed during this period of decreased intake (fig. 3).

Table 1. Anthropometric and physiological characteristics of the samples (mean ± SD)

	Weight, kg	Height, cm	VO_2max, ml/kg/min	% fat
Males				
Nonathletes	56.1 ± 6	166 ± 6 (244)	48 (21)	11.6
Athletes	54.6 ± 5	170 ± 4	72.5 (18)	9.2
Females				
Nonathletes	51.7 ± 6	155 ± 6 (280)	42 (12)	14.4
Athletes	50.5 ± 3	156 ± 5	60 (6)	12.8

Sample size (n) in parentheses.

Table 2. Mean energy intakes and nutrient composition

	Energy kcal/day	PR g/day	CHO g/day	Fat g/day	Animal PR g/day
Males					
Nonathletes	1954	58 (11)	380 (75)	30 (13)	5.2 (9)
Athletes	2340	62.5 (11)	441 (75)	36 (14)	8.1 (12.9)
Females					
Nonathletes	1672	49 (11)	329 (75)	25 (13)	4.1 (8.3)
Athletes	2017	60.4 (12)	374 (74)	31 (14)	7.5 (12.4)

The proportion in % is in parentheses.
kcal calculated roughly as fat, g × 9; CHO; g × 4; and PR, g × 4.

Table 3. Comparative energy intakes (kcal/day)

	FAO	Nonathletes	%FAO	Athletes	%FAO
Males	2,656	1,995	75	2,340	88
Females	2,242	1,713	76	2,017	90

n for M/F: nonathletes 214/214; athletes 18/6.

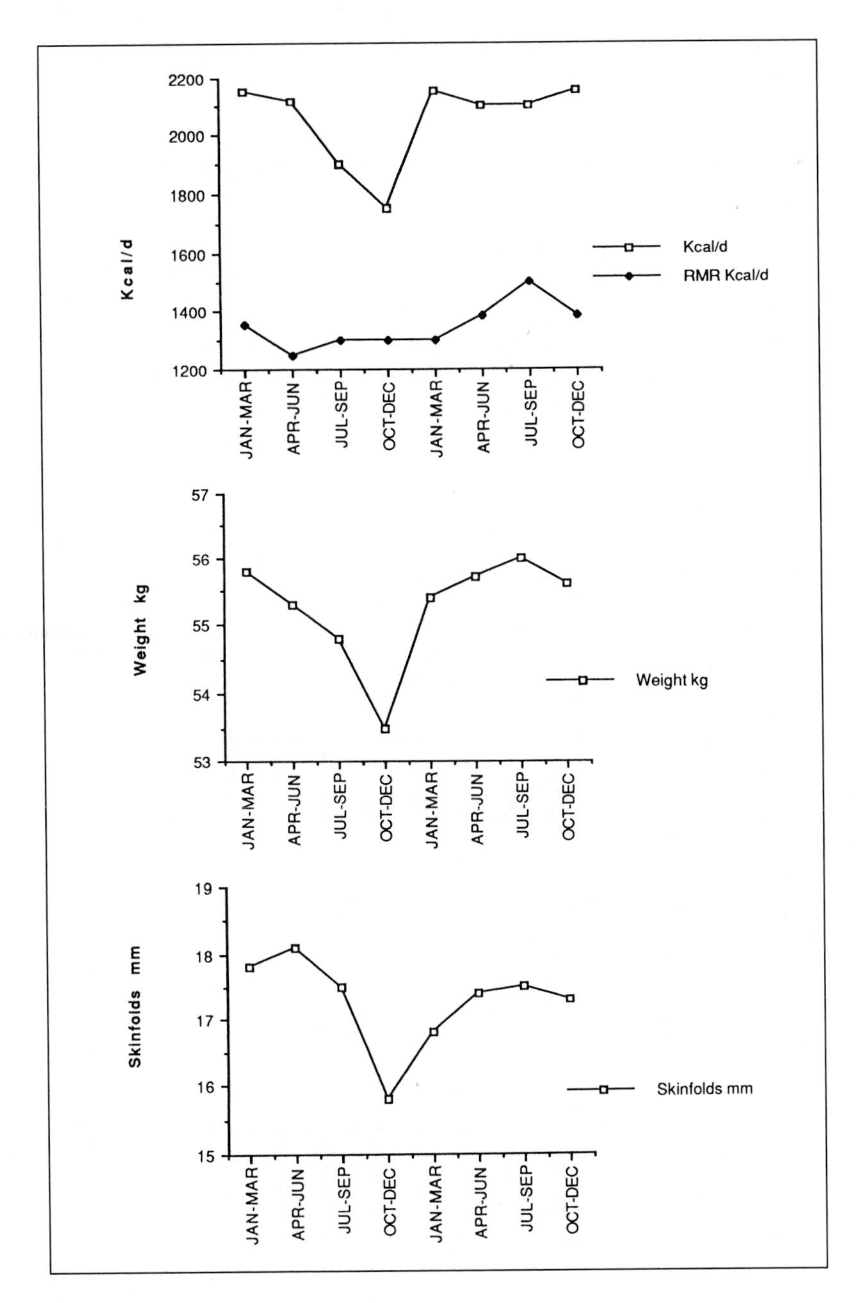

Fig. 1. Energy intake and RMR per day, body weight and sum of skinfolds for non-athletic males.

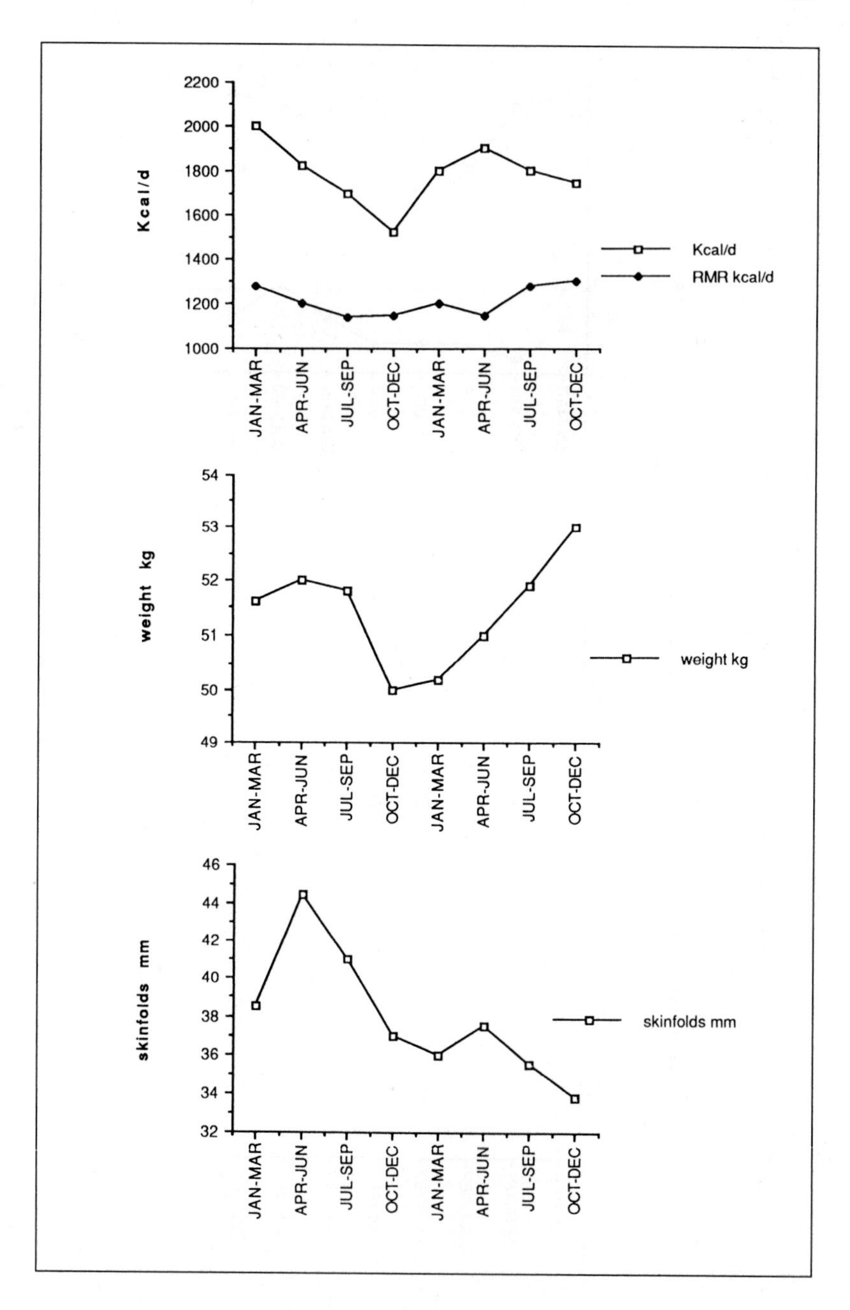

Fig. 2. Energy intake and RMR per day, body weight and sum of skinfolds for non-athletic females.

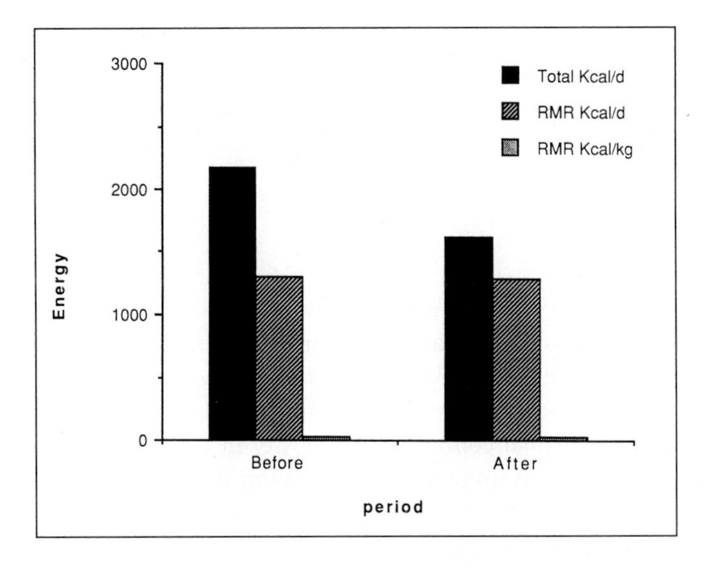

Fig. 3. Energy intake and RMR before and after the drought period.

Table 4. Iron intakes and iron indicators

	FE mg/d	Hb g/dl	Hct %	Ferritin mg/dl
Males				
Nonathletes	17.8	14.9	43.0	76
Athletes	22.4	15.0	43.5	72
Females				
Nonathletes	15.4	12.2	36.8	23
Athletes	15.8	12.6	37.1	24

Hematological parameters were evaluated to assess the impact of decreased energy and animal protein intakes (table 4), indicating no apparent decrements. Significant correlations were obtained between socioeconomic status (SES) and rice, wheat, milk, meat and fats (0.17–0.55) consumed. This indicates that these foods, though rarely consumed due to the cost factor, were in demand whenever income increased.

The most commonly consumed dishes are githeri (maize and kidney beans), ugali and sukumawiki (maize flour and kale), plantain/bananas, potatoes, millet and sorghum; clearly indicating a predominance of carbohydrates and legumes.

Discussion

In general a paucity of data exists on fitness and nutrition in Kenya. The aerobic capacities in the above groups are comparable to those reported in other populations [3]. Among the highly trained, the mean values have been replicated in tests done in other labs [Keul-Freiburg, Saltin-Karolinska, personal commun.]. Adiposity in both the nonathletic and athletic populations is quite low and is similar to previously reported values in farm workers in Kenya [4]. This may be attributed to lower energy intakes combined with an active lifestyle.

Overall, the total calorie intake is modest relative to established guidelines [5]. Although the measurement of food intake is subject to substantial error, we have tried to limit this by developing a nutrient database; a costly but necessary exercise to undertake. This involves investigation of existent data, accumulation of new data and validation of a resultant nutrient database [6]. Furthermore, during analysis of food composition of the typical dishes (multiple foods), the average difference between an actual dish and calculated components is less than 3%. However, underreporting may occur if there is social stigma associated with consumption of a food; for instance alcohol intake may not be readily acknowledged. On the other hand, since the diets contain large amounts of whole grain cereals, legumes and other plant foods high in fiber, which are less digestible, it appears in order that the figures of 4 kcal/g of carbohydrate (CHO) and protein (PR) and 9 kcal/g of fat obtained from the early 1900s need reconsideration.

A striking feature of the food intake proportions is the difference in fat, protein and carbohydrate intakes observed here and in other Kenyan populations [7] compared to elsewhere. Broadly speaking, the carbohydrate intake is much higher while protein and fats much lower as compared to intakes recommended in the west [8]. An interesting observation is that in Kenya, although the percentage of animal proteins was very low compared to other developing countries [2], there was no evidence that iron status was compromised in Kenyans even among the high-performance athletes. This should have worsened, especially since 30% of the population tested positive for malarial parasites, an anemia-causing agent [9]. Furthermore, no clinical signs suggestive of vitamin B or vitamin A deficiency were observed.

The period of food restriction provided an unexpected opportunity to examine the hypothesis that there is metabolic adaptation to chronic food restriction. Although weight loss occurred during this period, there was no evidence of adaptation through a decrease in resting metabolic rate. However, it is possible that activity patterns could have been, and probably were, less energy intensive during the drought.

Conclusion

After considering the many factors that could affect the validity of the energy intake and expenditure and their implications, the following conclusions seem warranted. Though total calorie intake and animal proteins were low, no vitamin B or A deficiencies were seen clinically. This emphasizes that RDAs are guidelines and that sometimes intake based on RDAs may be high in some populations. This is further elucidated by the observation that despite the low animal protein intakes, the plasma iron, hemoglobin and hematocrit levels were within normal limits. Furthermore, RMR was not lowered even with substantial decrements in total calorie intake.

As far as performance is concerned, an apparent inference is that a low total calorie intake does not necessarily deter performance if the meal is balanced and a high carbohydrate diet is consumed. Thus, in high-performance athletes, supplementation across the board needs further review. Athletes should be evaluated and supplemented on an individual basis. After all, 'more is sometimes better, sometimes worse and always costlier'.

One of the major problems in developing countries is that although there is a large volume of information available, this does not get to the target population. A practical solution to this dilemma would be to train the nutritionist/social worker to work with the target individuals, especially the mother. They should emphasize the 'balanced meal' concept rather than individual foods.

Secondly, malnutrition is primarily a socioeconomic problem – not enough to eat; therefore, to alleviate this malaise, it is imperative that the issue of unemployment/socioeconomic status be addressed as a long-term solution.

On the other hand, since there are a number of 'grey areas' in nutrition and fitness, donor countries could assist in setting up research centers in developing countries where these situations are already existent to collect and upgrade data bases in the fields of nutrition and fitness. Donors could assist in developing food strains with higher nutrient content as well as shorter growing periods per year. Finally, there should be re-emphasis (in economic packages) by donor groups on food crops and not only cash crops, since the former are important as reserve during crises. After all, a well-fed worker will always be more productive than one with malnutrition.

References

1 Thairu K: Fitness and nutrition policy in developing nations: Kenya's example. Am J Clin Nutr 1989;(suppl)49:1054–1056.

2 Food Intake and Human Function: A Cross-Project Perspective CRSP Program. Berkeley, University of California, 1988.

3 Astrand PO, Rodahl K: Textbook of Work Physiology. McGraw Hill, New York, 1986.

4 Prampero PE, Cerretelli: Maximal muscular power (aerobic and anaerobic) in African natives. Ergo 1969;12:51–59.

5 FAO/WHO/UNU Report of a Joint Expert Consultation on Energy and Protein Requirements: WHO Tech Rep Serv 724, Geneva, 1985.

6 Murphy SP, Weinberg SW, Andersson C, et al: Development of research nutrient data bases: An example using foods consumed in rural Kenya. J Food Composition Anal 1991;4:2–17.

7 Horweg J, Niemeyer R: Nutrition intervention research project, No 8: Report No 7, 1978.

8 Lemon PWR: Effect of exercise on protein requirements. J Sports Sci 1991;9(special issue):53–70.

9 Latham MC: Dietary and health interventions to improve worker productivity in Kenya. Trop Doctor 1983;13:34–38.

Meke Mukeshi, Department of Medical Physiology, Faculty of Medicine, University of Nairobi, PO Box 30197, Nairobi (Kenya)

Simopoulos AP (ed): Nutrition and Fitness in Health and Disease.
World Rev Nutr Diet. Basel, Karger, 1993, vol 72, pp 227–237

Some Recent Policies and Programs in Nutrition and Physical Fitness in China

Ji Di Chen

Research Division of Sports Nutrition and Biochemistry,
Institute of Sports Medicine, Beijing Medical University, Beijing, China

Introduction

China's economic reform and open policy have brought about rapid development of agricultural and industrial production, and there has been a steady increase in the production of major foods. As a result, consumption of major foods increased over the past 10 years (table 1) and the nutritional status of the population has significantly improved [1, 2]. According to the data of the Nationwide Nutrition Survey, energy intake was 2,845 kcal/day (RDA is 2,400 kcal/day), and protein 67 g/day (RDA 70 g/day) (table 2) [2].

Relevant to these changes, the incidence of some nutritional deficiency diseases such as scurvy and kwashiorkor have decreased or disappeared. In addition, improvement in growth and development of Chinese children has been significant. From 1975 to 1985, body height increased by 1.8 cm on average and weight increased by 0.4 kg for children 6–7 years of age. Average life span has increased from 35 years (1950) to 68 years (1988) [3]. However, nutritional insufficiencies are still common in rural areas. According to data from the Bureau of Statistics, in 1987 energy intake of 7.1% of peasants was less than 70% of the RDA. Nutrition intake of about 10% of the population was below the national average level. Calcium deficiency was common, energy from animal sources was only about 5% of the total intake, and the diet of peasants was mainly vegetarian [1, 3].

Although the general trend of body weight and height is gradually increasing, the prevalence of stunted and underweight children assessed as

Table 1. Consumption of energy and protein (1978–1987)

Year	Energy, kcal	Protein	
		g/day	% of total kcal
1978	1952	53	10.9
1980	2192	59	10.8
1982	2417	67	11.0
1984	2712	74	11.0
1986	2827	77	10.9
1987	2803	76	10.8
1982*	2485	67	10.8

Data from Chen [1].
* Data from 1982 Nationwide Nutrition Survey.

Table 2. % RDA of energy and protein (1978–1987)

Year	Energy, % RDA	Protein, % RDA
1978	81	76
1980	91	84
1982	101	95
1984	113	106
1986	118	110
1987	117	108
1982*	102	92

Data from Chen [1].
* Data from 1982 Nationwide Nutrition Survey.

height for age and weight for age of Chinese reference standards show that those below the 3rd percentile were 12.4–76.4% and 6.9–44.3%, respectively. Comparing the data with that of WHO showed that the height of Chinese children falls behind 5 and 10 cm for city and rural area children, respectively [4]. Investigation of 90,000 children from birth to 6 years of

Table 3. Anemia incidence of children of different ages from 1986 to 1989 (Hb < 110 g/l, n and %)

Age group years	1986		1987		1988		1989	
	n	%	n	%	n	%	n	%
<0.5	478	57.5	398	51.8	285	39.6	421	33.2
0.5–	704	62.3	709	60.2	725	54.2	760	51.0
1.0–	1,051	49.9	1,017	45.4	1,225	42.6	1,164	41.4
2.0–	908	37.7	831	33.7	1,149	28.3	1,083	27.5
3–5	1,929	28.4	1,961	25.8	2,576	18.8	2,283	17.6

Data from 'Child Nutrition Surveillance Working Team', 1990.

age illustrated that 10–20% of those investigated suffered from malnutrition [5]. About 15 million children were underweight. The incidence of rickets of those below 3 years of age was 30–50% and anemia was 30% (table 3) [3, 4]. Nutritional deficiency diseases are still prevalent in some parts of China and are important causes of ill health and premature death [3–5]. Thus, the main assignment is to further decrease the nutritional deficiency diseases, and improve the nutritional status of people and their health.

On the other hand, nutrition-related chronic diseases, attributed to incorrect balance or an excess of nutrient(s), are now of significant importance in some of the economically developed cities such as Beijing, Tienjin, and Shanghai, etc. Actually, these cities have already become 'aging cities'; chronic diseases such as cardiovascular, cancer, osteoporosis, and diabetes are rising and becoming the main causes of death [2, 6–8]. According to data from the statistics of the Ministry of Health, the death rate from chronic diseases accounted for 70% of the deaths (table 4).

Estimation of patients with chronic diseases in the whole country are as follows: high blood pressure, 60 million; diabetes, 15 million; cerebrovascular disease, 5 million.

In addition, there have been 1.3 and 1.2 million new patients with strokes and cancer, respectively, each year. Premature death caused by chronic diseases accounted for 63% of the loss of the nation's potential life span; and expenses for new patients reached up to 56 million yuan/year

Table 4. Death rate of the major diseases ($n/10^5$)

	City	Rural area
Cancer	141.34	112.79
Cerebral disease	120.07	102.55
Heart disease	78.10	74.12

Data from 'Study on Strategic Goals of Prevention at the year of 2000 at China', 1991.

which accounted for 3.3 times that of the funds for prevention for the whole city of Beijing.

The average calorie from fat intake of city residents contributed 29.5% of total calories in 1988, and 30% for Beijing and Tienjin residents. The incidence of overweight and obesity was as high as 50% in middle-aged and old women in 1987. The incidence of high blood pressure in 12- to 15-year-old adolescents reached 3,100/100,000 [6, 7]. Death induced by cardiovascular disease has risen from the 5th or 6th to the 1st or 2nd place. On the basis of calculations, the death rates for cardiovascular disease and cancer will be 3 and 2.6 times, respectively, those of the present by the year 2025 unless vigorous measures are adopted [3, 7]. Thus, emphasis on the prevention of chronic diseases is the immediate problem in order to protect health and decrease economic loss.

Nutrition Policies of the Chinese Government

To be fully aware of this fact, the Chinese government has taken measures and established policies concerned with the improvement of people's health and nutritional status.

(1) Work out a rational dietary pattern to provide principles for food planning and production and formulate dietary guidelines to guide people's eating habits and food choice for the prevention of both malnutrition and overnutrition.

On the basis of discussion over many meetings by scientists and government officials, and considering the nutritional needs of the population, capability of agricultural production, and potential of economic development of the country, a successful National Workshop on Dietary Guidelines for Food and Agriculture Planning was held in Beijing in 1989 where the participants put forward the following dietary principles for the Chinese people [1, 9].

(a) A national average daily energy intake of 2,400 kcal, with protein 70 g/day.
(b) Energy contribution from cereals, 60% of the total energy intake, and animal foods 14%.
(c) Protein intake from animal food and beans/pulses, 30–40% of the total protein intake.
(d) Energy intake from fat, 25–30% of total energy intake.
(e) Salt intake, less than 10 g/day.

Data from Chen [1].

With this dietary pattern, nutritional needs for people will be met, and the dietary quality will be improved and balanced. According to these principles, the annual per capita consumption of foods for the year 2000 was estimated; based on this, food production and food consumption goals in China for the year 2000 were also planned and estimated as follows [1]:

	kg/capita/year
Cereals	400
Oil seeds	21
Sugarcane and beets	88
Fruits	43
Meat	25
Eggs	12
Milk	15
Fish	14

Data from Chen [1].

However, the implementation of the dietary guidelines still will be a great challenge and will require tremendous effort because of such a large population of 1.25–1.3 billion by the end of this century, and due to limited land and the differences in economic, cultural and geographical conditions among different regions in China.

(2) For prevention and treatment of the main nutritional deficiency diseases such as iron deficiency anemia, rickets, and endemic goiter, the following measures already have been taken:

Table 5. The relative bioavailability of a series of iron preparations by Hb regeneration in rats

Iron preparations	RBA, %
Pig blood cell	73.9
Ferrous fumurate	114.9
Pig blood cell + ferrous fumurate compound	106.9
Marine alga iron	83.1
Tremella polysaccharide iron	74.3

RBA (relative bioavailability) of ferrous sulfate was used as a reference of 100%.

(a) Improve the quality of the diet.
(b) Apply foods with nutrient fortification.
(c) Treat existing patients.
(d) Establish monitoring systems gradually.

The Ministry of Health has supported a key research project for iron deficiency anemia by screening the oral iron preparations for relative bioavailability in rats. The results show that some of the organic iron preparations are helpful to patients with iron deficiency anemia (table 5). For treatment of patients with goiter, iodized salt has been handed out through prevention clinics.

(3) Guide people's consumption behavior to improve their nutritional status since consumption behavior not only influences nutritional status, but also makes rational use of the nation's resources.

(a) Spreading nutrition knowledge is a measure of great benefit with least investment. It is necessary to let people know the scientific reason for dietary guidelines. In recent years the Chinese people had to rely mainly on plant foods (grains, vegetables, etc.) whereas animal foods (meat, egg, poultry, milk, etc.) were subsidiary. On the basis of this principle, an adequate increase in animal foods and soybean or its products may guarantee sufficient nutrition and create a favorable situation for the prevention of overnutrition, and preventing risk factors for chronic diseases.
(b) Continue to carry out the rationing policy on grain and oil, etc.
(c) Control the price of rationed foods to guarantee the nutrition of the majority of Chinese people.

(d) Provide government subsidies for primary foods and living allowances; the subsidies should go up proportionally with food price. At present, efforts have been made to decrease the percentage of income used for food purchasing, and the Engel coefficient might decrease to $<50\%$.

(4) Establish a national nutrition monitoring system.

(a) Keep abreast of the Chinese people's nutritional status.
(b) Study the development of nutritional patterns and trends for change.
(c) Provide scientific information for planning government economics and health protection.

During 1985–1987, the Institute of Nutrition and Food Hygiene of the Chinese Academy of Preventive Medicine with the collaboration of seven provinces started activities on nutrition monitoring for preschool children. In 1990, under the support of WHO, FAO, and UNICEF, the Institute of Nutrition and Food Hygiene and the National Bureau of Statistics with the collaboration of provincial health institutions started to conduct tests at selected points to establish a nutrition monitoring system. It is estimated that 70% of the provinces and cities will establish nutrition monitoring systems in 1995, and these systems would carry out nutrition surveys and collect the data of weight and height of people for studying and improving their nutritional status [3].

Policies and Programs in China for Reduction of Nutrition-Related Diseases

Active measures have been adopted to decrease the risk factors of nutrition related diseases. Preventive work on nutrition related chronic diseases started rather late and the foundation is weak in China. Only some large cities carry out monitoring of cardiovascular and cerebrovascular patients. However, this has been put into China's Strategic Plan for the Year 2000, and it is estimated that the prevention-cure network will be organized soon [3, 7].

(1) Decrease salt intake and extend the use of low sodium foods.

WHO has stipulated the amount of sodium intake to be equivalent to 5 g of NaCl per day, but the average NaCl intake of Chinese people is much higher. The NaCl intake during 1982–1986 was 15–18 g/day for northern people, and 7–10 g/day for southern people. It has been found that the

Table 6. Epidemiological study on blood lipidiemia of middle-aged people with different nutrition

Indices	n	A	n	B
Age, years	61	49.8±6.2	981	49.4±8.3
BMI	61	24.8±2.5**	981	23.7±3.3
TC, mg/dl	61	215±54**	716	200±41
TG, mg/dl	61	114±31	716	128±72
High blood pressure, %	61	36.1	981	23.3

Group A were subjects with high protein and fat diet, and group B were subjects with a general Chinese diet.
** Comparison of the data between A and B group showed significant differences: $p < 0.05$.

Table 7. Planting area and production of soybean in China

Year	Planting area, 10,000 ha	Total production, 10,000 tons	kg/capita
1956	–	1,020	16
1957	1,275	–	–
1978	714	757v	<8
1987	845	1,218	11

Data from Liu [9]

incidence of high blood pressure was higher for people consuming >11 g/day NaCl than those of <11 g/day [7]. However, Chinese people have to adapt to a low salt diet and health education for the benefits of a low salt diet are needed. At the same time, stipulations should be provided for collective canteens, food companies and hotels; and production of low sodium foods is encouraged.

(2) Improve both the quantity and quality of dietary protein [10–13].

Since consumption of meat and eggs by the Chinese is increasing continously, there has been an increase of blood cholesterol levels. The investigation on blood lipids of a group of middle-aged people with high protein and fat diets showed that prevention measures should be taken urgently

Table 8. Vegetable consumption of Chinese in 1987

	Population, million	Average consumption, g/person/day
35 cities	0.56	250
Whole country	11.00	125

Data from Chen [11].

(table 6). Traditionally, Chinese eat more pork than other meats which accounts for about 80% of total meat. Experts appeal for a policy to increase production of soybeans to guarantee an annual supply of 13 kg/capita (table 7). Besides, increasing poultry production and strengthening the development of fish breeding are also important. The goal for aquatic and poultry products should reach 35–40% of total animal foods. In addition, price and subsidy should be favorably arranged.

(3) Control dietary fat intake.

Fat intake of people is closely correlated with the incidence and death rate from atherosclerosis. Calories from fat intake is increasing to more than 30% of the total intake in residents of large cities. Nutrition education about rational dietary composition is important to assist people to control dietary fat intake. The goal of dietary fat energy intake has been set at <28 and <20–25% of the total for city and countryside residents, respectively, in 1995; and it should be controlled to <30 and <25% for city and countryside residents respectively by the year 2000.

(4) Increase vegetable intake [14].

Vitamin A, B_2 and calcium insufficiency are common nutritional problems among the Chinese. Vegetables are the main sources for these nutrients. Development of vegetables is one of the most economic and effective measures. At present, average vegetable consumption is only about 200 g/day/person (table 8). Thus, it is of great importance to develop vegetable production in rural and remote areas, and efforts should be put in expanding vegetable resources. Although 17,000 kinds of vegetables are cultivated, there is still great potential for expansion.

A National Nutrition Guiding Committee has been approved by the Chinese government and was established in April 1992. Members of this committee include experts from agricultural, medicinal, nutritional, light industrial departments, and government officials. In order to supervise and improve people's health and nutritional status, this committee will consult on setting government nutrition policies, rules, management, and education, etc.

Nutrition as a discipline has been established in some of the medical universities which means that we will have more young nutritionists to carry on the nutrition work more actively in China in the near future.

Policies and Programs in Physical Fitness in China

(1) Carry out physical exercise among the mass of people to improve the quality of life and prevent chronic disease.

'Promote physical culture and build up people's health' has been the guiding principle since the establishment of New China. Policies to encourage people to participate in exercise are quite favorable. The government not only provides excellent nutritional conditions for elite athletes of training teams, but also pays a liberal subsidy for amateur athletes of sports schools, and for student athletes of general middle schools, colleges and universities. Physical training is an important course for students and is included as an important part of comprehensive education. Students who master excellent sports skills or reach elite athlete levels can have additional scores when enrolling into universities.

The Chinese government has acted vigorously to expand national or district games for people of different types of work and different ages, e.g. a National Game for Peasants and a National Game for Young People have been held in the past 2 years; in the near future the government will hold a National Game for Factory Workers and Staff Members.

Sports facilities have greatly improved, especially in large cities. Many new gymnasiums, tracks and fields, swimming pools, as well as a number of sports clubs including 'peace and happiness palaces' for exercise and recreational games, have been built in Beijing, Guangzhou, Chengdu, etc.

In addition, mass organizations of provincial and city sports federations have taken the initiative to organize a variety of exercise activities such as summer camp, weight reduction courses, aerobic dancing (Chinese Tai-Ji and Jian-Mei) courses, and nutrition counseling programs for parents and aged people on vacation, etc. These activities assist and attract millions of people to join into more exercise and liven up cultural and recreational activities.

From the point of view of managing preventive activities for chronic diseases, departments of health care also actively organize people to join into exercise, e.g. pilot projects on high blood pressure management have been launched in Beijing and Tienjin which include advocating adequate exercise.

References

1 Chen CM: Dietary CM: Dietary Guidelines for Food and Agriculture Planning in China. The Compilation of International Symposium on Food, Nutrition, and Social Economics Development. Beijing, China Science & Technique Publishing House, 1991, pp 34–48.

2 Jing DX, Chen CM, et al: Summary of the Whole Nation's Nutrition Investigation. The Institute of Nutrition and Health, China Academy of Preventive Medicine, 1985, pp 53–76.

3 Child Nutrition Surveillance Working Team: The Nutritional Status of the Preschool Children in Some Poor Areas in China. The Compilation of International Symposium on Food, Nutrition, and Social Economics Development. Beijing, China Science & Technique Publishing House, 1991, pp 64–69.

4 Chen JS: Contrasting Nutrition Experiences in the East and West. Presented at the 6th Asian Congress of Nutrition, Kuala Lumpur, September 17, 1991.

5 Chen JS: Changes of Disease Model and the Countermove Direction of Prevention and Treatment. Chin Prevent Med 1990;24:290–292.

6 Zhao FJ: Studies on the Relationship between Dietary Composition, Health and Disease. The compilation of International Symposium on Food, Nutrition, and Social Economics Development. Beijing, China Science & Technique Publishing House, 1991, pp 86–91.

7 Chinese Nutrition Society: The dietary guidance of the Chinese. Acta Nutr Sin 1990; 12:10–12.

8 Mei FQ, Tao ZS, Li ZQ: An analysis of the trends in China's food development to the year 2020. The Compilation of International Symposium on Food, nutrition, and Social Economics Development. Beijing, China Science & Technique Publishing House, 1991, pp 123–128.

9 Liu JX: To Increase Animal Food in Chinese People's Diet. Beijing, China Science & Technique Publishing House, 1991, pp 164–168.

10 Li OU, Li XY, Jian XY: An Approach to Increasing the Meat Production in China: Tentative Plan of Establishing Modern Cattle Indusry Systems in Northern China. Beijing, China Science & Technique Publishing House, 1991, pp 200–204.

11 Chen H: The Potential Improvement of Human Nutrient by Vegetable Crops. Beijing, China Science & Technique Publishing House, 1991, pp 210–214.

Ji Di Chen, MD, Research Division of Sports Nutrition and Biochemistry, Institute of Sports Medicine. Beijing Medical University, Beijing 100083 (China)

Subject Index